Diffuse Malignant Mesothelioma

Timothy Craig Allen
Editor

Diffuse Malignant Mesothelioma

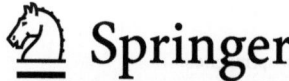

Editor
Timothy Craig Allen
Department of Pathology and Laboratory Medicine
The University of Texas Medical Branch
Galveston
Texas
USA

ISBN 978-1-4939-2373-1   ISBN 978-1-4939-2374-8 (eBook)
DOI 10.1007/978-1-4939-2374-8

Library of Congress Control Number: 2014960083

Springer New York Heidelberg Dordrecht London
© Springer Science+Business Media New York 2015
This work is subject to copyright. All rights are reserved by the Publisher, whether the whole or part of the material is concerned, specifically the rights of translation, reprinting, reuse of illustrations, recitation, broadcasting, reproduction on microfilms or in any other physical way, and transmission or information storage and retrieval, electronic adaptation, computer software, or by similar or dissimilar methodology now known or hereafter developed.
The use of general descriptive names, registered names, trademarks, service marks, etc. in this publication does not imply, even in the absence of a specific statement, that such names are exempt from the relevant protective laws and regulations and therefore free for general use.
The publisher, the authors and the editors are safe to assume that the advice and information in this book are believed to be true and accurate at the date of publication. Neither the publisher nor the authors or the editors give a warranty, express or implied, with respect to the material contained herein or for any errors or omissions that may have been made.

Printed on acid-free paper

Springer New York is part of Springer Science+Business Media (www.springer.com)

*To my parents, Oliver and Mildred, my wife
Fran, and my daughters Caitlin and Erin.*

Preface

Many thanks to the authors who spent countless hours in researching and writing their chapters on the various aspects of diffuse malignant mesothelioma. Their hard work and support in developing and writing this book was invaluable.

This book is meant to be a straightforward resource for issues basic to the diagnosis of diffuse malignant mesothelioma. Moreover, and importantly, the book is meant to present an unbiased examination of diffuse malignant mesothelioma; The editor has not testified nor worked as an expert witness, and at the time of writing and editing this book does not plan to testify or otherwise work as an expert witness, in lawsuits involving the diagnosis of diffuse malignant mesothelioma, either for plaintiffs' attorneys or for defendants' attorneys.

T. C. Allen

Contents

1. **Approaching the Diagnosis of Diffuse Malignant Mesothelioma** 1
   Timothy Craig Allen

2. **Epidemiology** 3
   Lynette M. Sholl and Marina Vivero

3. **Clinical and Radiologic Features** 33
   Anja C. Roden and Christine U. Lee

4. **Histology** 69
   Mahmoud Eltorky

5. **Immunohistochemistry** 93
   Nahal Boroumand

6. **Molecular Characteristics** 107
   Grace Y. Lin

7. **Therapy** 125
   Eric Bernicker, Puja Gaur, Snehal Desai, Bin S. Teh
   and Shanda H. Blackmon

Index 141

Contributors

Timothy Craig Allen Department of Pathology and Laboratory Medicine, The University of Texas Medical Branch, Galveston, TX, USA

Eric Bernicker Cancer Center, Houston Methodist Hospital, Houston, TX, USA

Shanda H. Blackmon Department Thoracic Surgery, Houston Methodist Hospital, Houston, TX, USA

Nahal Boroumand Department of Pathology, University of Texas Medical Branch, Galveston, TX, USA

Snehal Desai Department of Radiation Oncology, Houston Methodist Hospital, Houston, TX, USA

Mahmoud Eltorky Department of Pathology, University of Texas Medical Branch, Galveston, TX, USA

Puja Gaur Department Thoracic Surgery, Houston Methodist Hospital, Houston, TX, USA

Christine U. Lee Department of Radiology, Mayo Clinic, Rochester, MN, USA

Grace Y. Lin Department of Pathology, UC San Diego Health System, San Diego, CA, USA

Anja C. Roden Department of Laboratory Medicine and Pathology, Mayo Clinic, Rochester, MN, USA

Lynette M. Sholl Department of Pathology, Brigham and Women's Hospital and Harvard Medical School, Boston, MA, USA

Bin S. Teh Department of Radiation Oncology, Houston Methodist Hospital, Houston, TX, USA

Marina Vivero Department of Pathology, Brigham and Women's Hospital and Harvard Medical School, Boston, MA, USA

Chapter 1
Approaching the Diagnosis of Diffuse Malignant Mesothelioma

Timothy Craig Allen

For most pathologists, diffuse malignant mesothelioma (DMM) is a disease for which its rarity renders it unfamiliar, its histologic diversity diagnostically challenging, and its medical–legal implications overly stressful. Because DMM has a dismal prognosis and very limited treatment options compared to its much more common mimics, accurate diagnosis is paramount.

The World Health Organization's classifications of tumors of the pleura [1] and peritoneum [2] include DMM; however, as the vast majority of DMM is pleural, it is pleural tumor upon which this book focuses. DMM is the most common primary malignant neoplasm arising within the pleura. The WHO's classification also recognizes four DMM histologic subtypes: epithelial, sarcomatous, biphasic, and desmoplastic; however, the designation of desmoplastic DMM—generally considered a variant of sarcomatous DMM—as a separate histologic subtype is controversial. Although desmoplastic DMM is strongly mimicked by chronic fibrous pleuritic, and has an especially bad prognosis, neither of these features warrants the stature of independent subtyping.

In order to render an accurate diagnosis, a biopsy sample must provide adequate diagnosable tissue. For the diagnosis of DMM, such a biopsy sample typically is obtained from open procedures such as thoroscopy. Pleural needle biopsies have the benefit of low morbidity and cost; however, those efficiencies often come at the high cost of diagnostic compromise [3, 4]. Once determined adequately, a tissue sample must then be assessed to determine whether it contains reactive or neoplastic tissue, and if neoplastic, whether the tumor is DMM or another, likely metastatic, neoplasm. The differential diagnosis and workup are guided by the histology, specifically by the presence of an epithelioid cellular proliferation or a spindle cell proliferation. In these cases, even with ample tissue available for examination, histology alone is typically insufficient to allow a definitive DMM diagnosis to be rendered, and im-

T. C. Allen (✉)
Department of Pathology and Laboratory Medicine, The University of Texas Medical Branch, 301 University Blvd., 2.190JSA, Galveston, TX 77555, USA
email: timallenmdjd@gmail.com

munostains are a necessary next step in the diagnostic workup. Yet immunostains themselves also have significant limitations; for example, their use in determining reactive versus neoplastic tissue is very restricted, and their utility with spindle cell proliferations is also narrow. Further, it must be remembered that both neoplastic and reactive proliferations may be present in a single biopsy. *En face* sectioning might also show sheet-like collections of mesothelial cells suggesting the presence of a solid tumor. Also, nuclear atypia involving reactive proliferations may be so marked as to mimic malignancy, while DMM may present with generally bland-appearing nuclear features. In the end, numerous potential diagnostic pitfalls must be avoided. Ultimately, biopsy findings must be correlated with clinical and radiologic findings to best ensure accurate diagnosis.

DMM is frequently associated with prior occupational exposure to asbestos; however, asbestos exposure history is irrelevant to the histologic diagnosis of DMM, or its exclusion from a differential diagnosis, and should not be used as a factor in the histologic diagnosis of DMM. A misdiagnosis may yield substantial medical–legal consequences.

Because DMM diagnosis—and often even its mere clinical speculation—initiates legal proceedings, pathologists—subject to resultant diagnostic pressure—must maintain the highest level of professionalism and diagnostic accuracy. It must be remembered that the vast majority of cases for which DMM is clinically entertained in the end are either reactive proliferations or metastases. To best serve the patient, consultation with a pulmonary pathologist with expertise in DMM diagnosis is recommended in all but the most straightforward of DMM cases. One should reasonably assume that the pathologist's DMM diagnosis will be carefully scrutinized in the legal arena.

References

1. Travis WD, Brambilla E, Muller-Hermelink HW, et al. Pathology and genetics of tumors of the lungs, pleura, mediastinum and heart. Lyon: IARCPress; 2004.
2. Tavassoli FA, Devilee P. Pathology and genetics of tumours of the breast and female genital organs. Lyon: IARCPress; 2003.
3. Boutin C, Rey F. Thoracoscopy in pleural malignant mesothelioma: a prospective study of 188 consecutive patients. Cancer. 1993;72:389–3.
4. Attanoos RL, Gibbs AR. The comparative accuracy of different pleural biopsy techniques in the diagnosis of malignant mesothelioma. Histopathology. 2008;53:340–4.

Chapter 2
Epidemiology

Lynette M. Sholl and Marina Vivero

Introduction

Malignant mesothelioma is defined by the World Health Organization (WHO) as a malignant neoplasm arising from mesothelial cells and growing in a diffuse pattern over the surfaces lining body cavities, including pleura, peritoneum, pericardium, and tunica vaginalis [1]. In approximately 90% of cases, malignant mesothelioma arises in the pleura, where it is often diagnosed at a late stage and associated with relatively rapid death [2]. A causal link between asbestos exposure and malignant mesothelioma was first drawn in studies published in the 1960s [3]; this association has since been confirmed in diverse populations across the globe in relation to both occupational exposures and naturally occurring forms of environmental asbestos. Currently, the WHO recognizes asbestos as an important occupational carcinogen and has committed to an initiative to eliminate asbestos-related diseases globally [4].

Incidence of Pleural Mesothelioma

Epidemiologic studies from the early 2000s estimated that mesothelioma is responsible for 43,000 deaths a year worldwide [5] at a mean age of 70 [6], and is more common in industrialized countries [2]. However, in light of the difficulties in diagnosing this tumor type, it has been estimated that for every four individuals diagnosed with malignant mesothelioma, another one goes undiagnosed [7]. In fact, the absence of robust disease reporting practices in countries with known asbestos consumption patterns has led some authors to speculate that approximately 39,000 cases went underreported between 1984 and 2008 in Russia and east, south, and

---

L. M. Sholl (✉) · M. Vivero
Department of Pathology, Brigham and Women's Hospital and Harvard Medical School,
75 Francis Street, Boston, MA 02115, USA
e-mail: lmsholl@partners.org

© Springer Science+Business Media New York 2015
T. C. Allen (ed.), *Diffuse Malignant Mesothelioma*, DOI 10.1007/978-1-4939-2374-8_2

central Asia [7]. Analysis of the global impact of mesothelioma is complicated by several factors, including variable reporting practices in different countries, the lack of an International Classification of Diseases (ICD) code specific to malignant mesothelioma prior to 1993, and variable accuracy worldwide in diagnosing cause of death [6]. Further, in reporting periods spanning the 1990s and early 2000s, the assessment of anatomic site-specific incidence rates was confounded by the fact that nearly half of all cases were reported as arising at "unspecified sites"; however, the available data do suggest that pleural disease is about ten times more frequent than mesothelioma arising at other sites [6].

Worldwide, the incidence of malignant mesothelioma has been rising since the mid-twentieth century, with the best-documented increases in diagnoses noted in Australia and the UK. The most recent data from the UK suggest a fivefold increase in the incidence in men between 1980 and 2009, with an annual incidence of 29 per million [2]. Based on usage patterns of asbestos-containing materials in the twentieth century, peak incidence in many developed countries is expected to occur in the second and third decades of the twenty-first century [8–11]. Despite declarations from the WHO and other international organizations to halt the use of asbestos in manufacturing and construction, developing countries, especially those in Asia undergoing rapid industrialization, continue to use asbestos, and thus are expected to see further growth in the incidence of malignant mesothelioma [12].

The USA Surveillance, Epidemiology, and End Results (SEER) program data collected by the National Cancer Institute documents an incidence of 12.5 per 100,000 among US men and 2.3 per 100,000 among US women over 65 years of age. The incidence of mesothelioma increases steadily with age in men (Fig. 2.1). White non-Hispanic men are at highest risk of disease, with an overall nationwide incidence rate of 2.2 per 100,000 (irrespective of age), as compared to 0.6, 1.1, and 1.6 per 100,000 Asian/Pacific Islanders, Blacks, and Hispanics, respectively [13]. The incidence of mesothelioma varies from state to state, with the highest rates noted in Louisiana, New Jersey, and Seattle–Puget Sound in the 2005–2009 time period [13]. This regional clustering reflects the presence of local industries that have historically used asbestos, including shipbuilding, petrochemical manufacturing, and refining [2]. Likely as a result of regulatory efforts and declining use of the more carcinogenic amphibole forms of asbestos in US manufacturing practices (see below), the incidence of mesothelioma in US men that peaked in the early 1990s has declined consistently since that time [14] (Fig. 2.2).

Risk Factors for Malignant Pleural Mesothelioma

Malignant pleural mesothelioma is highly associated with asbestos exposure. A study examining populations derived from Los Angeles, New York State, and Veterans Administration Hospitals nationwide estimated that the attributable risk for exposure to asbestos among men with pleural mesothelioma was 88% [15]. The risk of pleural mesothelioma following exposure to asbestos is dose dependent, as clearly documented in the Wittenoom cohort of crocidolite miners and millers

2 Epidemiology

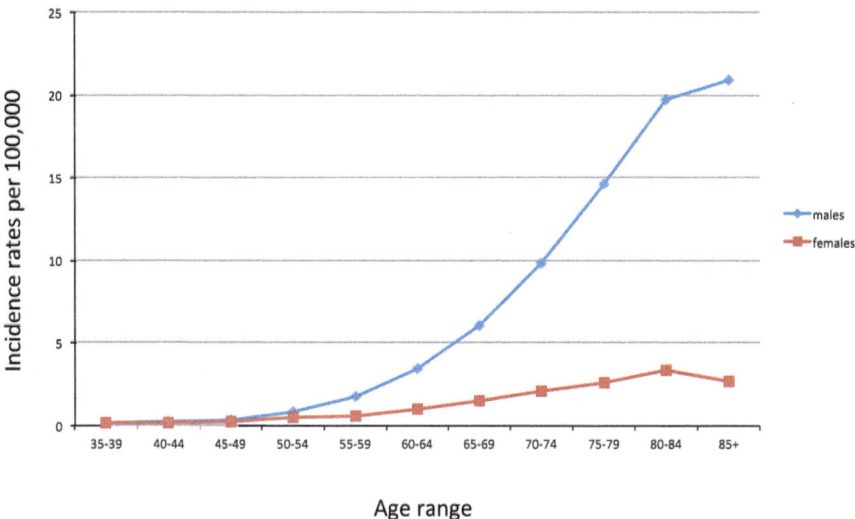

Fig. 2.1 Age-adjusted rates of malignant mesothelioma in the USA according to gender. (Adapted from SEER data)

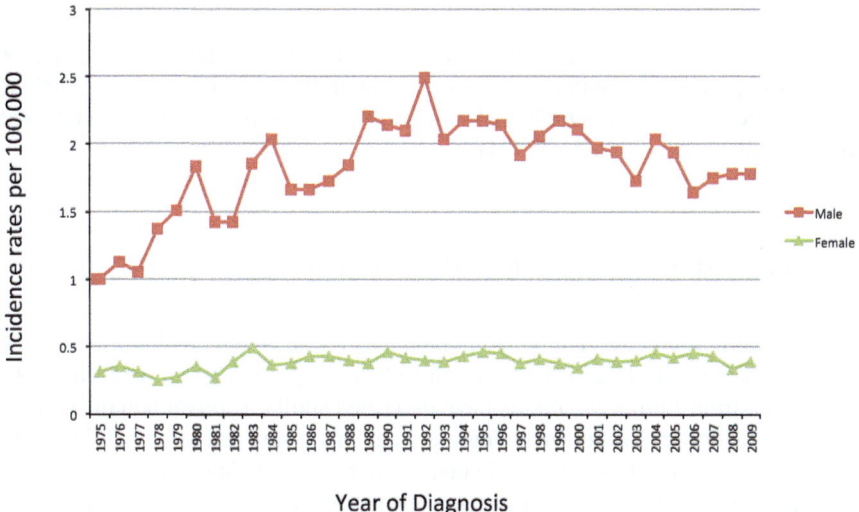

Fig. 2.2 Age-adjusted SEER incidence rates of mesothelioma from 1975–2009 according to gender

from Western Australia [16]. Risk increases in a linear or supralinear fashion over time, even after exposure cessation [17]. The clinical presentation of mesothelioma lags behind the time of first exposure by about 30 years (latency period). Thus, the increasing incidence of pleural mesothelioma in the 1970s reflected a surge in asbestos usage in war-related manufacturing during World War II, and the peak incidence of pleural mesothelioma in the USA in the early 1990s reflects the peak use of amphiboles in US manufacturing practice in the 1960s [18]. Worldwide, men are three- to fourfold more likely to die of malignant pleural mesothelioma than women [6]. This observation reflects higher likelihood of more intense asbestos exposure among men than women in post-World War II industrial practice. Studies of women engaged in the manufacture of crocidolite-containing gas masks in England during World War II showed that they too were at significantly increased risk of death from lung and pleural tumors as compared to other malignancies [19].

Environmental exposure to asbestos poses an increased, albeit generally lower risk as compared to occupational exposure, with family members of asbestos workers and those who live in proximity to asbestos industries showing an increased risk for pleural mesothelioma as compared to other geographic cohorts [20]. Remarkably, high frequencies of pleural mesothelioma have been documented in rural populations where asbestos is present in surface soil and residents have long-standing environmental exposure to the fibers. One cohort study of the rural Dayao community in southwestern China, where crocidolite is prevalent in the soil, estimated an annual mesothelioma mortality rate of up to 365 per million, with mesothelioma accounting for 22% of cancer deaths [21]. Studies from southeastern Turkey have documented a two- to fivefold increased incidence of malignant pleural mesothelioma among inhabitants of villages where soil-containing tremolite and chrysotile have been used for whitewashing and other household purposes, as compared to villages where asbestos-containing minerals have not been detected [22, 23]. Even in the absence of direct exposure to asbestos-containing soil related to farming or household practices, proximity to sources of naturally occurring asbestos, such as serpentinite and other ultramafic rocks in California, is associated with an increased risk of malignant mesothelioma [24].

Prognosis of Malignant Pleural Mesothelioma

As of the mid-2000s, survival in US populations for all comers with mesothelioma was 40.9% at 1 year, 12.2% at 3 years, and 3.9% at 5 years [13]. More recent population data from European cohorts have described similar survival outcomes, with adverse prognostic features including older age, male sex, and sarcomatoid histology [25, 26]. Current use of multimodality therapy, including surgery, radiation, intracavitary chemotherapy, and systemic chemotherapy, has led to some improvement in survival, but these approaches are rarely curative and are controversial [27]. Retrospective analysis of population-based data derived from the SEER dataset of patients diagnosed with malignant mesothelioma demonstrated no significant improvement in overall outcomes over the past four decades, with a median survival of 7.2 months for patients diagnosed in the 1970s versus 7.1 months in the 2000s [13] (Fig. 2.3). There has been a statistically significant improvement in survival among patients with distant disease (5.5 months in 1970s versus 7.0 months in 2000s, $p=0.001$); however, this improvement is marginal in clinical terms [28].

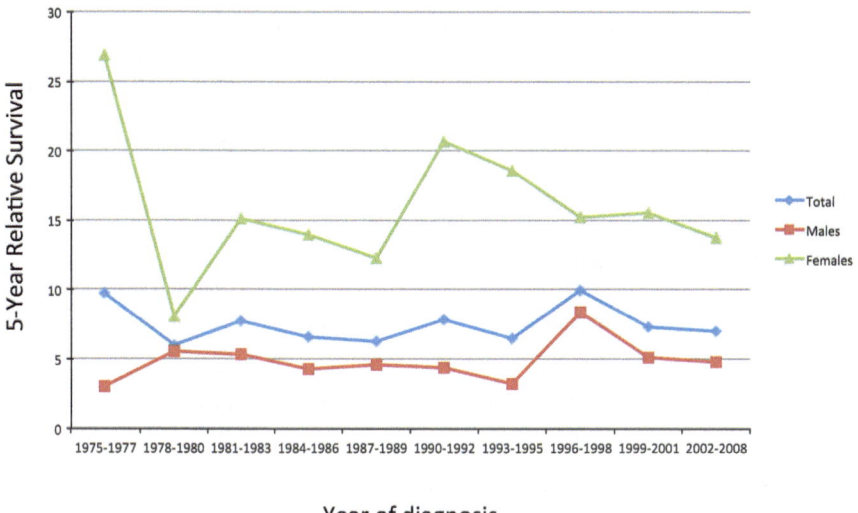

Fig. 2.3 A 5-year relative survival of patients with mesothelioma by gender and year of diagnosis

In patients undergoing chemoradiotherapy and/or surgery, features associated with adverse survival include male gender, sarcomatoid histology, and advanced pathologic stage according to the American Joint Committee on Cancer staging system [29, 30].

Asbestos and Malignant Mesothelioma

A substantial body of literature is dedicated to the physical and chemical features of asbestos fibers that contribute to carcinogenesis. The results of these studies have resulted in a widely accepted "fiber pathogenicity paradigm" encompassing the characteristics of a pathogenic fiber and the general process by which it leads to tumor formation. In general, a fiber must (a) be inhaled, (b) travel through the upper respiratory tract and be deposited in the lower respiratory tract, (c) persist within the body for a significant amount of time, (d) travel to the parietal pleura, and (e) possess pro-inflammatory and genotoxic physical and chemical properties. In vitro, in vivo, and human epidemiologic studies of asbestos and other fibers have suggested that fibers with high-aspect (length-to-diameter) ratios of >3:1, small diameters (0.25–0.4 µM), and longer fibers with a minimum length of 5 µM (ideally, lengths of >10 µM) produce the greatest pathogenic effects [31–36]. Fibers possessing these qualities are present in significant quantities in many widely used types of asbestos and asbestiform materials, and are thought to account for the majority of fiber-related malignant pleural mesotheliomas [35, 37]. While the physical properties of fibers are thought to mediate most of their carcinogenic effects, the chemical

Table 2.1 Asbestos fiber types, carcinogenic potency, and commercial uses

Fiber	Mineralogic group	Potency	Commercial use
Chrysotile (serpentine)	Chrysotile	Low	Cement, textiles, friction products
Crocidolite (Riebeckite)	Amphibole	High	Pipe production, gas masks, cigarette filters[a]
Amosite (Cummingtonite/Grunerite)	Amphibole	Intermediate	Cement, textiles, insulation[a]
Anthophyllite	Amphibole	Limited data	Construction, insulation Contaminant of talc
Tremolite	Amphibole	Limited data	Contaminant of crysotile, talc, vermiculite, diamond mines
Actinolite	Amphibole, chemically similar to tremolite	Limited data	Gemstones (jade, cat's eye); co-contaminant with tremolite

[a] Historical uses only in most industrialized countries

composition of a pathogenic fiber is also contributory inasmuch as it affects fiber structure, ability to generate oxidative damage, and biopersistence.

The principal types of commercial asbestos are chrysotile, amosite, and crocidolite, also known as white, brown, and blue asbestos, respectively, based on their physical coloration (Table 2.1). Amosite and crocidolite are amphiboles, according to their mineralogic properties. Industries in which workers are most likely to be exposed to one of these forms of asbestos include mines, textile industries, and manufacturing of cement, insulation, and brakes (Table 2.2). Of these three fiber types, crocidolite is associated with the highest risk of mesothelioma development; risk of death from mesothelioma following crocidolite exposures is up to one order of magnitude higher than following amosite exposure and two orders of magnitude higher than with chrysotile exposure [38].

Chrysotile is the most commonly employed asbestos fiber, historically accounting for ~95% of total asbestos use [39]. The pathogenicity of chrysotile fibers in development of mesothelioma has been up for debate. Studies of lung tissue from Quebec miners and millers with mesothelioma have demonstrated that very-high-fiber loads of chrysotile can be oncogenic in the absence of significant concentrations of amosite or crocidolite. However, in many cases, chrysotile is accompanied by high levels of tremolite, particularly in mining and textile industries, thus the actual etiologic agent is unclear [40]. Indeed, chrysotile fibers, unlike the amphiboles, are not readily retained in the lung. Chrysotile is relatively fragile and fragments easily, permitting phagocytosis by pulmonary macrophages, and may actually dissolve in lung tissue due to leaching of magnesium out of the fiber. In contrast, amphiboles (which include tremolite) have a straight and broad structure and do not fragment readily, thus they are less susceptible to phagocytosis, and are chemically stable in a biologic environment [41].

Table 2.2 Occupations associated with pleural and peritoneal mesothelioma

Anatomic site	Occupation[a]
Pleural	Insulation
	Asbestos production and manufacture
	Plumbing
	Vehicle body building
	Shipbuilding/shipyard/ship repair
	Construction
	Furnace/boiler installation and repair
	Brake lining work
	Building demolition
	Production of paper products
Peritoneal	Insulation
	Asbestos production and manufacture
	Vehicle body building
	Construction
	Plumbing
	Cement workers
	Mining

[a] Occupations are listed in order of approximate highest to lowest risk

Anthophyllite, actinolite, and tremolite are less commonly used in industrial practices in the USA, although these have been mined and used for commercial purposes in other countries and are known contaminants of other industrial minerals including talc and vermiculite. Studies in animal models have suggested that anthophyllite is carcinogenic and contributes to the development of malignant mesothelioma [42]; however, confirmed human cases of anthophyllite-attributable mesothelioma are very rare [43]. Tremolite is a contaminant of other mineral deposits, including chrysotile (see above) and vermiculite, which is used as a form of insulation and a gardening material. In addition to the epidemiologic evidence linking environmental exposure to tremolite in Turkish villages to malignant mesothelioma (see above), occupational exposure to tremolite is linked to development of disease as well. Cohort studies from Libby, Montana, the location of a large tremolite-contaminated vermiculite mine, have shown that miners, millers, and processors of vermiculite were significantly more likely to die of asbestos-related diseases, including mesothelioma, than the general population [44]. Actinolite is chemically similar to tremolite and may be found in combination with tremolite deposits, but is less common [45].

Irrespective of these different chemical and biologic properties, all of these fibers are classified together for the purposes of defining workplace regulations under the Occupational Safety and Health Administration (OSHA) [46] and are regulated under the Environmental Protection Agency's Clean Air Act [47]. The Toxic Substances Control Act banned manufacture and importation of asbestos-containing paper products and flooring felt, as well as any nonhistorical, "new uses" of asbestos.

The Clean Air Act and Consumer Product Safety Act have banned the use of materials containing >1% asbestos that are sprayed on and asbestos-containing wall-patching compounds [48].

In the USA, asbestos-containing products persist in construction, clothing, and car manufacture and repair [47]. Chrysotile was used in automotive brakes until its use was banned by the Environmental Protection Agency (EPA) in the 1980s. Although OSHA cites an unspecified risk of mesothelioma among automotive mechanics, epidemiologic studies to date have failed to demonstrate an increased incidence among this group relative to background [49]. Similarly, chrysotile was ubiquitous in industrial and residential drywall products until the late 1970s; despite some reports of asbestos-related disease among individuals who used drywall-patching compounds, subsequent epidemiologic studies failed to confirm any health risks associated with using these products. A recent study of Chinese chrysotile-textile plant workers demonstrated an excess risk of lung cancer and respiratory diseases, although the small number of individuals included in the study precluded drawing any conclusions with regard to risk of mesothelioma [50].

Mesothelioma and Non-Asbestos Fibers

Almost all studies concerning non-asbestos fibers as etiologic agents in malignant pleural mesothelioma are based on the assumption that any natural or man-made fiber that fits the "fiber pathogenicity paradigm" (see above) has carcinogenic potential in humans (Table 2.3).

Biogenic Silicates in Plant Fibers

The presence of silica and silicates in asbestiform fibers and the observation of increased lung cancer and mesothelioma risk in Louisiana and Indian sugarcane farmers with no known asbestos exposure led to an investigation of silica fibers in sugarcane [51, 52]. Certain plants have been shown to absorb and accumulate environmental silica, yielding, according to Newman et al., needle-shaped biogenic crystals of approximately 0.85 µM in diameter and 10–300 µM in length [51]. Although additional epidemiologic studies of farming-related fiber exposure have not been performed, the theoretical risk of mesothelioma associated with biogenic silica crystals has been proposed based on their physical similarity to asbestos fibers.

Erionite

Erionite is a naturally occurring non-asbestos fiber. Records of mesothelioma "epidemics" in small villages of central Anatolia in Turkey, where mesothelioma

Table 2.3 Strength of evidence for increased risk of mesothelioma in non-asbestos exposures

Agent	Mode of exposure	Strength of evidence
Radiation	Iatrogenic	Strong
SV40 Infection	Contaminated polio vaccines	Insufficient
Natural fibres		
Erionite	Environmental/building material	Strong
Fluoro-edenite	Environmental	Limited
Plant-derived silicates	Occupational	Insufficient
Man-made fibres		
Glass wool[a]	Insulation	Insufficient
Continuous glass filaments[a]	Textiles, plastics	Insufficient
Rock and slag wool[a]	Thermal and acoustic insulation	Insufficient
Refractory ceramic fibers[a]	High-temperature insulation	Insufficient
P-aramids	Insulation, automotive products	Insufficient
Carbon nanotubes	Occupational	None

[a] Based on conclusions made by the International Agency for Research on Cancer (IARC) Monographs Working Groups in 2001

accounts for up to 50% of mortality, began to surface in 1975 and 1978. Examination of rock and dust samples from the area in 1979 demonstrated the presence of erionite fibers <0.25 µM in diameter and up to 5 µM in length, and spurred continued study of the natural fibers and epidemiology of mesothelioma in the region. Baris et al. conducted a survey of the Anatolian villages of Karain, Karlik, and Sarihidir in 1987, demonstrating that respirable erionite fibers composed 20–80% of dust clouds in the village streets and that higher levels of exposure correlated with increased mortality from mesothelioma [53]. In vitro and in vivo inhalational studies in rodents have confirmed the potent carcinogenicity of erionite, which has been listed as a group I known human carcinogen by the International Agency for Research on Cancer (IARC) working group [54–56]. Environmental studies in the USA have identified naturally occurring erionite in North Dakota, South Dakota, Nevada, Oregon, and other areas of the western USA, and have demonstrated physical similarities between the erionite fibers present in those locations and those known to cause mesothelioma in Turkey [56, 57]. One small published series demonstrated radiologic changes in erionite-exposed North Dakota residents similar to those seen in asbestos-exposed individuals [57], and a single case report of erionite-associated mesothelioma in the USA [58]; however, more epidemiologic studies will be necessary to determine the erionite-associated cancer burden in the USA.

Other Natural Fibers

Exposure to fluoro-edenite, another natural fibrous amphibole first detected in eastern Sicily, has been shown to correlate with the risk of mesothelioma in patients with no known asbestos exposure in one small case series [59].

Synthetic Fibers

Synthetic organic and inorganic fibers have been produced in greater quantities worldwide as a response to increased regulation of asbestos, and are used in a variety of industrial and domestic products. Inhalational studies in animals have revealed sufficient evidence to suggest that special-purpose glass fibers and refractory ceramic fibers have significant carcinogenic potential, but only limited evidence of carcinogenicity pertaining to other inorganic fibers [60]. There is some evidence of dose-dependent radiographic pleural and interstitial changes in populations exposed to inorganic synthetic fibers, usually occurring 15–20 years after exposure, but these results are frequently confounded by asbestos and smoking exposure, and limited by small numbers of patients. Overall, epidemiologic studies of workers exposed to inorganic man-made fibers have not shown significant increases in mortality due to pleural malignancy in comparison with unexposed populations [60–62].

P-aramids, a type of organic man-made fiber used in heat-resistant fabrics, ropes, cables, brake pads, and other products, have been studied in animals and shown to have mild pro-inflammatory, pro-fibrotic, and proliferative effects on the pleura, but have not been shown to cause mesothelioma [37]. No human cases of malignant or nonmalignant disease have been documented as a result of p-aramid exposure.

Carbon Nanotubes

Carbon nanotubes (CNTs) are cylindrical or bundle-like man-made carbon structures with properties that potentially fit the fiber pathogenicity paradigm [35, 36]. Animal studies have demonstrated that intraperitoneal, intratracheal, and inhalational exposure to CNTs results in increased inflammation and fibrosis [35, 63, 64]. Consistent with the fiber pathogenicity paradigm, long CNTs appear to be more pathogenic than short CNTs. Mesothelioma has been reported in *Trp53* heterozygous mice and in wild-type mice following peritoneal and scrotal injection with CNTs [64], but additional studies will be necessary to draw definitive conclusions about the risk of mesothelioma in CNT-exposed animals and humans. No documented cases of mesothelioma in humans exposed to CNTs currently exist.

Malignant Pleural Mesothelioma and Simian Virus 40

Simian virus 40 (SV40) is a virus of Asian macaques generally thought not to be infective in humans unless artificially introduced. Large-scale human exposure to SV40 occurred between 1956 and 1966 in areas of Europe, Great Britain, and the USA as a result of widely-distributed contaminated polio vaccines grown in monkey renal-cell cultures. Approximately 10–15% of selected populations who were not exposed to the contaminated vaccine are reported to be seropositive for SV40, however, suggesting that other routes of human infection may exist [65, 66]. Interest in the association between SV40 infection and mesothelioma oncogenesis originates from observations in the 1960s that SV40 is oncogenic in rodents and from a study by Cicala et al. in 1993 indicating that intrapleural, intraperitoneal, or intracardiac injection of live SV40 induces pleural or peritoneal mesothelioma in 70% of exposed hamsters [67]. In vitro studies suggest that malignant transformation of SV40-infected cells is a rare event and likely depends on the integration of SV40 DNA into the host genome. Proposed mechanisms of carcinogenesis include chromosomal damage via SV40 integration into the host genome, suppression of p53 and Rb by the SV40 large T antigen (Tag), and other direct effects of Tag [68, 69].

The role of SV40 in the development of human mesothelioma has been a topic of controversy over the past two decades. The majority of the positive evidence for SV40 oncogenicity in mesothelioma lies in the detection of SV40 DNA, RNA, or protein in patient tumor samples or the finding that SV40 is capable of altering cell proliferation and immortalizing cells in vitro. SV40- or SV40-like sequences have been detected in up to 60% of frozen and paraffin-embedded mesothelioma samples, and immunohistochemical and western blot evidence of SV40 Tag expression in tumor tissues has been reported [68, 70, 71]. A synergistic effect between SV40 exposure and asbestos exposure on the risk of developing mesothelioma has also been proposed in humans [71]. Other studies, however, have failed to demonstrate significant amounts of SV40 DNA or RNA sequences in tissue samples, including those collected from patients known to be seropositive for SV40 [72–74]. Geographic variation in SV40 exposure has been proposed to account for the variability of results among studies. Other explanations for the variability of results in the literature have been posited. Significant sequence and antigenic overlap exist between SV40 and other papovaviruses that do commonly infect humans, including the John Cunningham (JC) and BK viruses. In addition, SV40 sequences found in commonly used laboratory plasmids may result in polymerase chain reaction (PCR) contamination and false-positive results. Pepper et al. amplified SV40 sequences in six of nine mesotheliomas by PCR; however, all SV40-positive cases were also positive using a broader primer set that amplified a sequence common to the BK, JC, and SV40 viruses [75]. Lopez-Rios et al. subsequently performed a systematic study of 71 mesotheliomas and found that 62% of cases were positive by PCR using SV40 primers that amplify sequences also found in commonly used laboratory plasmids, 23% were positive using plasmid-specific primers, and only 6% were positive for natural SV40 sequences not known to exist in laboratory plasmids [76]. Some serologic studies in mesothelioma patients using different techniques have suggested a slightly increased, although not always significant, prevalence of SV40 seropositivity in mesothelioma patients compared with control patients, but have also demonstrated inter- and intra-study variability, and the results do not reliably correspond to the presence of SV40 in matching tumor tissue [65, 73, 74].

Epidemiologic evidence of a relationship between SV40 and increased incidence of mesothelioma has not been established, due to the fact that the only definitively proven route of human SV40 infection is administration of contaminated vaccines, and it is often impossible to accurately determine individual vaccination exposure status. Vaccine contamination rates, furthermore, have varied from 10 to 100% in different countries and in selected populations, making it even more difficult to estimate true SV40 exposure rates [68, 77, 78]. Epidemiologic studies failing to demonstrate association between SV40 exposure and mesothelioma typically examine patient cohorts who are younger than the expected median age of patients with mesothelioma; however, most SV40 exposure is thought to occur in the first few years of life and the follow-up times in many of the largest epidemiologic studies of SV40 and mesothelioma have reflected the expected 30–40-year latency period for mesothelioma development following asbestos exposure. While a few studies have found increased incidence of mesothelioma in populations potentially exposed to contaminated polio vaccine, the results have not reached statistical significance [68]. Strickler et al. found no significant increase in mesotheliomas or other cancers among exposed US populations, but the study was limited by a small patient population [79]. Studies examining cancer incidence in highly exposed populations (86–95% of all Danish children born between 1955 and 1962 were exposed to contaminated lots of vaccine) have also failed to demonstrate a relationship between SV40 exposure and mesothelioma [78]. Other large studies in the USA and UK have similarly failed to show a consistent relationship between potential SV40 exposure and the development of mesothelioma [66, 77].

Radiation-Associated Mesothelioma

Exposure to external beam radiation has been reported as a risk factor for the development of secondary mesothelioma in the context of treatment for a variety of malignant and nonmalignant conditions, primarily Hodgkin and non-Hodgkin lymphoma, breast cancer, and testicular tumors [80–89]. Most reports consist of single cases and small series, and suggest that radiation-associated mesothelioma occurs within the radiation field after doses ranging from approximately 20 to 90 Gy, affects men and women at equal rates, and has a prognosis similar to asbestos-associated mesothelioma of the same histologic subtype. Reported latency between exposure and development of secondary pleural malignant mesothelioma has ranged from 5 to 41 years after radiation exposure [82].

Many existing studies examining the association between radiation exposure and mesothelioma are limited by small patient cohorts, inadequate information regarding radiation dose, and failure to address occupational history or asbestos exposure. A 20-year review of 1000 recipients of thoracic radiation performed in 1995 at a major cancer center uncovered three instances of presumed secondary malignant mesotheliomas, suggesting a higher incidence compared with the general population, but did not provide further information regarding latency periods, radiation dosages, prognosis, or demographic features [90]. A study published in 1996 examining nearly 1.5 million patients registered in the SEER database reported 33 radiation-associated malignant mesotheliomas [82]. Patients in this cohort were treated for a variety of thoracic, abdominal, and pelvic malignancies, had a median age of 68.5 years, latency of 4.3 years, and sex distribution similar to asbestos-related mesothelioma. Tumors occurred most frequently in patients treated for prostate, colon, and breast cancers. This study, however, included patients who developed mesothelioma within 2 months after primary diagnosis, and, importantly, did not address asbestos exposure as a possible confounder.

Subsequent studies have primarily looked at specific populations of patients (i.e., patients treated for breast cancer, Hodgkin lymphoma, etc.) using updated data from the SEER program and nationwide registries in Norway, Sweden, Finland, Denmark, the Netherlands, and Germany [91–97]. Taking into account all studies that exclude patients who develop mesothelioma within 2 months of primary tumor diagnosis, latency from exposure to diagnosis is 16–28 years, the median reported survival of radiation-associated mesothelioma is approximately 10 months, and sex distribution is similar to that of asbestos-related tumors. Epithelioid histology appears to predominate, and only in rare instances have mixed or sarcomatoid histology been described. The relative risk of mesothelioma in radiated patients with no history of asbestos exposure generally falls in the range of 1.42–3.74 but has been reported to be as high as 19.5. Multiple factors have been proposed to alter the relative risk of developing mesothelioma and account for the variability between studies, including the type of primary cancer, sex, age at radiation, and synergistic effects of asbestos or chemotherapy exposure. DeBruin et al., for example, reported a markedly increased relative risk of 44.8 in patients who received chemotherapy in addition to radiotherapy; however, this effect has not been noted in other studies [92]. Hodgson et al. studied secondary cancers in nearly 19,000 5-year survivors of Hodgkin lymphoma and reported a significant effect of sex and age at radiation in the development of multiple secondary cancers, including mesothelioma, with female patients radiated at ages younger than 20 possessing the greatest 30-year cumulative risk [94].

Thorotrast, a solution of thorium dioxide that emits α, β, and γ radiation, was used as an imaging contrast medium throughout Europe and the USA during the 1930s and 1940s. After use during angiography, thorotrast persists in the body, becomes concentrated in the reticuloendothelial system, and has been linked to malignancies of the liver, kidney, and bone marrow, among others. The earliest report of an association between thorotrast exposure and mesothelioma described a malignant mesothelioma of the "cervical pleura" in a 43-year-old woman, 25 years after extravasation of thorotrast, during an imaging procedure, but did not define diagnostic criteria or offer a description of the tumor [98]. Subsequent larger studies have confirmed significantly elevated risks of mesothelioma in patients with both systemic and localized exposure to thorotrast in comparison to unexposed patients, despite the smaller relative doses (Gy) of radiation compared to those used during treatment of malignancy [99].

Analyses of individuals with occupational and environmental radiation exposure have suggested some increased risk of mesothelioma as compared to similar populations without known exposure to radiation, but are confounded by concurrent asbestos exposures [99, 100].

Familial Malignant Pleural Mesothelioma

Evidence of a genetic predisposition for the development of mesothelioma is derived primarily from reports of familial clustering, and more recently, observation of syndromic associations, whole-exome sequencing, and genome-wide association studies.

Familial Clustering of Malignant Pleural Mesothelioma

Studies of "familial malignant pleural mesothelioma" are all limited by small sample sizes and are generally confounded by the presence of asbestos exposure in study subjects, including indirect exposure via spousal or parent–child interactions, which has been reported to confer up to a tenfold increased risk of developing malignant pleural mesothelioma [101]. Inaccurate estimates of exposure levels, limited availability of medical records, and inability to confirm the diagnosis of mesothelioma in older studies also prompt caution in interpretation of the results. Nevertheless, several families with multiple cases of malignant pleural mesothelioma have been described, supporting an argument for the presence of some genetic predisposition. The first familial cluster of malignant mesothelioma was described in 1965, and interest in the possible genetic basis of the disease rose steadily during the 1980s as other familial cancer predisposition syndromes were discovered. Risberg et al. described one of the largest familial aggregates of mesothelioma to date in a two-generation study of a family in which a father, three sons, and daughter succumbed to either peritoneal or pleural mesothelioma [102]. Affected family members died in their sixth and seventh decades, were all smokers, and had minimal-to-mild asbestos exposure. Similar subsequent studies have described aggregates of two to four family members with pleural and peritoneal mesotheliomas [103–106]. While some small series report a significantly younger mean age at presentation in affected individuals, overall there have been no significant differences observed in age, gender, histologic subtype, latency, duration of asbestos exposure, or distribution of disease between familial and sporadic mesotheliomas [103, 107]. A few studies have looked at lung asbestos fiber content in familial mesotheliomas and have yielded variable results, further adding to the uncertainty regarding the role of asbestos exposure in these cases [104, 105].

Larger studies of familial clusters of mesothelioma have been carried out in special populations with a higher baseline incidence of mesothelioma. de Klerk et al. analyzed 20 families from Wittenoom Gorge in Western Australia who had been involved in asbestos milling between 1943 and 1966 and in which at least two members were affected by malignant pleural mesothelioma [108]. The findings suggested a doubled risk of mesothelioma in blood relatives of affected family members, compared to no increased risk in spouses who had married into the families, the latter finding contrasting with previous reports regarding indirect exposure [101]. The risk of developing mesothelioma in these families was influenced by the duration of asbestos exposure and age at first exposure. A similar study in the

Trieste–Monfalcone area of Italy, an area with a history of asbestos milling, revealed clustering of mesotheliomas among 19 families with 40 affected individuals, all of whom had had variable levels of asbestos exposure [109].

Additional studies have examined the populations of Karain and Tuzkoy, two small villages in Turkey in which up to 50% of mortality is due to erionite-associated mesothelioma. Although genealogy has been difficult, Roushdy-Hammady et al. performed thorough kinship mapping in an initial study of these two towns based on verbal reports, town records, and medical records, which revealed a number of families with clusters of up to four affected family members per generation, including spouse, parent–child, and sibling pairings [110]. Overall, 50% of each generation in these families was affected by mesothelioma, with a median age at death of 55 years and a male-to-female ratio of 1.26. Comparison of erionite exposure and fiber composition between houses belonging to affected and unaffected families revealed no differences. Furthermore, surveys of 300 immigrants to Sweden and 250 immigrants to Germany from Karain and Tuzkoy, respectively, showed a similar incidence of mesothelioma compared to town members who did not emigrate. This combination of findings was interpreted as evidence of a genetic predisposition to the development of mesothelioma that is inherited in an autosomal-dominant fashion among families in Karain and Tuzkoy. This suggestion has been challenged on the basis of inaccurate methods of collecting data, a high baseline incidence of mesothelioma in these towns, high levels of erionite exposure among study subjects, and the fact that women who married into "mesothelioma families" also developed mesothelioma [111].

Studies based in Sarihidir, another Turkish village with a high incidence of mesothelioma, confirmed variable interfamily incidence of mesothelioma, despite equivalent estimated levels of erionite exposure [112]. Individuals who married into affected families and developed mesothelioma also originated from "mesothelioma families," and Carbone et al.'s report indeed notes that few people from surrounding villages married or moved into Karain and Tuzkoy villages, suggesting a limited local gene pool and lending support to the argument for genetic predisposition in this population [113]. In contrast to earlier reports, however, no mesotheliomas were detected among 24 descendants of affected families who were raised outside of Sarihidir; however, all patients were aged 26–46 and therefore younger than the median age of affected individuals [112]. Other authors studying Karain have concluded that genetic predisposition does not play a role in the incidence of mesothelioma in these communities based on the similar risk of developing mesothelioma between immigrants into and out of the village and the fact that the only variable that correlated with increased risk for mesothelioma was the duration of time spent living in Karain [114]. It is notable, however, that the incidence of mesothelioma among immigrants to Karain was nevertheless much lower than that in residents of Karain, and that the follow-up time of emigrants from Karain in this study may not have been sufficient to make definitive statements about the incidence of mesothelioma in this population. On balance, available studies of these communities do suggest that the development of mesothelioma is the product of interaction between genetic predisposition and environmental exposure.

Genetic Associations

A number of theories have surfaced to explain the genetic mechanisms for predisposition to mesothelioma, including deficiencies in subsets of T cells, natural killer cells, abnormalities in the *PDGFRB* gene, deficiencies in superoxide dismutase, and various human leukocyte antigen (HLA) associations; however, none of these factors have reliably been associated with increased incidence of mesothelioma [107, 115, 116]. The finding that up to 41 % of sporadic mesotheliomas possess mutations in the *NF2* gene also raises the possibility that individuals with germ-line *NF2* mutations might have a predisposition to develop mesothelioma, and while animal studies have suggested that this may be the case, reports of mesothelioma in neurofibromatosis patients are restricted to rare case reports [117–119].

Extensive study of individuals with N-acetyltransferase 2 (*NAT2*) and glutathione S-transferase M1 (*GSTM1*) mutations has been pursued after initial reports suggested that individuals with inactivating mutations in these genes were more susceptible to developing mesothelioma [120]. Hirvonen et al. compared 44 Finnish mesothelioma patients to 270 controls and determined that 61 % of mesothelioma patients versus 46 % of controls had a *GSTM1* null phenotype, 68 % of mesothelioma patients had a *NAT2* slow-acetylation phenotype versus 51 % of controls, and that the group of patients with abnormalities in both genes had a threefold incidence of mesothelioma compared with patients who had none [120]. These findings, however, were only marginally significant, and subsequent studies have similarly only found a marginal or variable association between abnormalities in these genes and incidence of mesothelioma [116, 121].

Two series have suggested some association between abnormalities of *XRCC1* and *ERCC1* DNA repair genes and mesothelioma in an Italian population exposed to asbestos, but this association remains to be confirmed [121, 122].

Two genome-wide association studies have revealed several gene polymorphisms associated with higher risk of mesothelioma in Italian and Australian populations, including in *MMP14, THRB, SDK1, FOXK1,* and *CRTAM* among others [118, 123]. There was, however, little overlap in associations when the two populations were compared, with the exception of the region of 7p22.2 flanking the *SDK1* gene; it is unclear if the polymorphisms identified have causal significance or if they are in linkage disequilibrium with other unidentified risk alleles.

BAP1 Syndromic Disease

Loss-of-function nonsense and truncating mutations in the BRCA1-associated protein 1 (*BAP1*) gene were identified in two Wisconsin families with a high prevalence of mesothelioma and no known exposure to asbestos or erionite [124]. Nearly a quarter of sporadic mesotheliomas harbors somatic loss of function mutations in *BAP1,* and a small but appreciable number of patients with apparently sporadic disease have germ-line mutations in *BAP1* [124, 125]. Using sequencing, fluorescence in situ hybridization (FISH), and immunohistochemistry, the prevalence of mutation, copy number loss, and/or protein expression loss in BAP1 in mesothelioma primary samples and cell lines ranges from 18–42% [125]. Biallelic somatic *BAP1* alterations are common in malignant pleural mesothelioma, and are detected in up to 60% of cases, by some accounts [126, 127].

Germ-line *BAP1* mutations are associated with an autosomal-dominant pattern of hereditary mesotheliomas in association with a syndrome consisting of familial mesothelioma, uveal melanoma, cutaneous melanoma, and distinctive epithelioid melanocytic tumors [128, 129]. Other tumors, including renal, lung, breast, colorectal, thyroid, and prostate malignancies have also been reported in individuals with germ-line *BAP1* mutations [130, 131].

Peritoneal Malignant Mesothelioma

Many of the epidemiologic associations pertaining to malignant pleural mesothelioma also apply to malignant mesothelioma arising in the peritoneum. There are, however, several important site-specific differences in the demographic features, genetics, and distribution of histologic subtypes between mesotheliomas arising in the pleura and peritoneal cavities that suggest fundamental biological disparities between tumors at these sites. The most pronounced difference between pleural and peritoneal mesothelioma is the higher prevalence of indolent histologic variants and lower prevalence of sarcomatoid mesothelioma in the peritoneum, both of which potentially affect the epidemiology of peritoneal disease.

Diagnostic Categories

Diffuse peritoneal malignant mesotheliomas are categorized into epithelioid, sarcomatoid, and mixed subtypes, the most common being the epithelioid type. Tumors of mixed subtype have been reported to comprise from 5 to 22% of peritoneal malignant mesotheliomas, although some mixed tumors were likely placed in the epithelioid category in certain studies, making it likely that the percentage of mixed cases is closer to 20% and therefore only slightly lower than the estimated prevalence of 30% in the pleural cavity. Pure sarcomatoid morphology, in contrast, is extremely rare in the peritoneum, and is estimated to comprise 2% or less of peritoneal mesotheliomas, compared to approximately 10% of malignant pleural mesotheliomas [132–134].

Diffuse peritoneal malignant mesotheliomas should be distinguished from other distinctive forms of peritoneal mesothelioma, including the indolent and often incidentally identified well-differentiated papillary mesothelioma and the so-called benign multicystic mesothelioma. Both of these latter entities are, in stark contrast to diffuse malignant mesothelioma, strikingly more common in women, with well-differentiated papillary mesothelioma reported at a male to female ratio of 6:1 in some studies [135, 136]. These tumors occur at a younger median age and are in most cases associated with a benign course, with only a few deaths attributable to either disease in the published literature. There is no clear association between these forms of mesothelioma and asbestos exposure; however, both well-differentiated papillary mesothelioma and benign multicystic mesothelioma have been associated with prior surgery or inflammatory conditions such as endometriosis [137, 138].

General Epidemiology

Incidence

Malignant peritoneal mesothelioma accounts for 10–20% of all mesotheliomas, with approximately 250 newly diagnosed cases in the USA each year [139]. An overall incidence in the general population of about 0.5–3 cases per million persons per year has been estimated based on information from population-based registries in the USA and Europe [140–142]. Teta et al. have reported a slightly higher incidence in men of 1.1 cases per million, compared to 0.6 cases per million women, confirming the male to female incidence ratio of approximately 2:1 seen in smaller series [142].

Risk Factors

Occupational asbestos exposure is the primary recognized risk factor for the development of diffuse malignant peritoneal mesothelioma and is present in an estimated 33–52% of cases [139, 143, 144]. The precise relationship between asbestos exposure and peritoneal malignant mesothelioma, however, is not yet fully understood and does not appear to be entirely analogous to the relationship with pleural disease. Although some studies suggest a dose-dependent increase in peritoneal mesothelioma upon asbestos exposure, the occupations that correlate with high rates of malignant pleural mesothelioma do not fully overlap with those that confer an increased risk of peritoneal disease [145, 146]. Spirtas et al.'s study of 25 peritoneal mesotheliomas has also suggested a differential effect of asbestos exposure in men and women, with no significant correlation between exposure and disease in women, although very few female patients were included in the study [144]. Other more uncommon etiologic factors in malignant peritoneal mesothelioma are discussed below.

Demographics

Peritoneal malignant mesothelioma is more common in men than women, with reported male to female ratios varying from 13:1 in asbestos-exposed populations to

1.6–2:1 in unselected populations [6, 132–134, 140, 147]. However, peritoneal malignant mesothelioma comprises a greater proportion of mesotheliomas in women, accounting for approximately 22 % of total mesotheliomas in women, compared with 11 % in men [141, 142]. This distribution of disease in women has been interpreted to indicate that occupational exposure is less important in peritoneal disease than it is in pleural disease, but this hypothesis remains unproven.

Prognosis

Median survival of malignant peritoneal mesothelioma patients in studies that exclude well-differentiated papillary mesothelioma and benign multicystic mesothelioma has varied, likely due to small sample sizes, but generally shows little difference in overall survival compared to pleural malignant mesothelioma. Large studies carried out in the USA, Italy, and Germany suggest an average overall survival of approximately 10–13 months [139, 143]. A few patients selected for aggressive cytoreductive therapy and perioperative chemotherapy have been reported to have median survivals of up to 67–79 months after diagnosis [147, 148].

Of note, despite the lack of statistically significant differences in survival, several groups have reported a greater proportion of long-term survivors in malignant peritoneal mesothelioma than in pleural disease, and report that women tend to have a more favorable prognosis, particularly after treatment [143, 145, 148]. Some studies have demonstrated that women are significantly more likely to have less extensive and lower stage disease than men, thus suggesting that women develop less aggressive tumors [145, 148]. The histologic inclusion criteria are not clearly delineated in many such studies, however, and it is likely that they are contaminated by cases of the biologically distinctive forms of disease more common in women—benign cystic mesothelioma and well-differentiated papillary mesothelioma.

Mortality Rates

A survey of mesothelioma mortality in the USA between the years 1999 and 2007 performed by the Centers for Disease Control's National Institute for Occupational Safety and Health revealed 657 deaths due to peritoneal disease, accounting for 3.6 % of total mesothelioma deaths in the USA [149]. Of note, only 8.3 % of mesothelioma deaths in this study were attributed to pleural disease, and approximately 75 % of the death certificates reviewed did not specify anatomic site, making it possible that these data do not represent the true proportion of mesothelioma deaths due to peritoneal disease in the USA. Analysis of the WHO mortality database, which included 83 countries, revealed an age-adjusted mortality rate of 0.3 per million per year for peritoneal mesothelioma and showed that 4.5 % of mesothelioma deaths between 1994 and 2008 were due to peritoneal disease, compared with 41.3 % due to pleural disease [6].

Non-Asbestos Fibers and Peritoneal Malignant Mesothelioma

Erionite

Direct intrapleural or intraperitoneal injection of erionite, as well as inhalational exposure, has been shown to induce diffuse malignant peritoneal mesothelioma in animal models, but may not necessarily reflect the levels of exposure or pathogenic mechanism of erionite in humans [150]. A few small series examining residents or immigrants from the Turkish villages of Karain, Tuzkoy, and Sarihidir, where up to 50% of mortality is due to erionite-related malignant mesothelioma, have mentioned rare cases of peritoneal mesothelioma, which appears to account for 7–14% of mesotheliomas in these villages [53, 114, 151]. While the numbers of patients with malignant peritoneal mesothelioma in these studies are small, the combination of data from animal studies and increased incidence of disease in erionite-exposed populations, in the context of the rare occurrence of disease in control populations, strongly suggests a pathogenic role for erionite in malignant peritoneal mesothelioma.

Synthetic Fibers

Several animal studies have shown that intraperitoneal injections of glass wool, other special-purpose glass fibers, rock wool, and ceramic fibers may result in mesothelioma [60]. No human cases of peritoneal mesothelioma due to synthetic fiber exposure have been published.

Carbon Nanotubes

Intraperitoneal injection of CNTs into rats has been shown to cause peritoneal fibrosis and inflammation in wild-type mice, but has not been shown to cause mesotheliomas in animal studies, with the exception of a single study suggesting carcinogenic potential in p53 mutant mice [63, 64, 152]. No human cases of mesothelioma related to CNT exposure have been reported.

Peritoneal Malignant Mesothelioma and Simian Virus 40

Simian virus 40 infection has been suggested as a possible etiologic factor for pleural mesothelioma, and intraperitoneal injection of live SV40 into mice and hamsters has been shown to result in malignant peritoneal mesothelioma [67]. Almost all investigation of SV40 in human mesotheliomas, however, has focused on pleural disease, thus little is known regarding SV40 and peritoneal malignant mesothelioma. Although PCR-based studies have identified a high rate of SV40 large T antigen positivity in small series of peritoneal malignant mesotheliomas [153], larger epidemiologic studies of SV40 in peritoneal mesothelioma are lacking. At this time, any conclusions about a significant role for SV40 in peritoneal mesothelioma must be drawn from analogy with pleural disease, which has shown no significant population-wide association with SV40 exposure.

Radiation-Associated Peritoneal Malignant Mesothelioma

Radiation-associated peritoneal malignant mesothelioma, like radiation-associated malignant pleural mesothelioma, has generally been reported to occur in the direct field of radiation for germ cell tumors, cervical cancer, and Hodgkin lymphoma. Additional case reports and small series have suggested a lag time of 13–31 years after radiation exposure, with a survival ranging from 9 to 24 months from the time of diagnosis, and predominantly epithelioid morphology [81–83, 88]. One case of peritoneal mesothelioma in a radiation technologist has also been reported [82].

In 1975, Maurer and Egloff first described malignant peritoneal mesothelioma after pericholecystic thorotrast extravasation during an imaging procedure, occurring as a mixed epithelioid and sarcomatoid tumor in a 48-year-old woman with a lag time of 36 years [154]. Subsequent population-based studies in Danish, German, Swedish, Japanese, and US populations have found a higher incidence of peritoneal malignant mesothelioma in patients exposed to systemic thorotrast exposure during cerebral or limb angiography compared with similar but unexposed patient populations [99, 155, 156]. One report noted one peritoneal malignant mesothelioma among 370 patients, prompting the conclusion that the low levels of peritoneal radiation exposure attributable to systemic use of thorotrast did not result in mesothelioma; however, the small patient population and presence of an otherwise rare tumor is nevertheless notable. The numbers of peritoneal malignant mesotheliomas in these studies have been low, but the cumulative findings suggest a relationship to both localized and systemic thorotrast exposure.

Familial Peritoneal Malignant Mesothelioma

Familial Clustering

Familial clustering of peritoneal malignant mesothelioma has been described in several mesothelioma families that are also affected by malignant pleural mesothelioma, suggesting that a possible genetic predisposition to both pleural and peritoneal disease may exist [102, 104, 105, 157]. While not all familial clusters include both pleural and peritoneal disease, reports of isolated familial peritoneal mesothelioma are rare; however, whether these differing mesothelioma "phenotypes" actually signify a different underlying genetic basis of disease is unknown. Interestingly, many reports that specifically address isolated familial peritoneal mesothelioma and specify histologic variants appear to most commonly describe benign multicystic mesothelioma, possibly suggesting a hereditary tendency to form this specific subtype of mesothelioma [158, 159].

Overall, familial peritoneal malignant mesothelioma appears to arise at a similar age and has a similar prognosis to sporadic peritoneal malignant mesothelioma, but appears to comprise a smaller proportion of familial mesothelioma in women [103]. These findings are based on a small number of cases however, and may not truly represent the clinical features of familial peritoneal malignant mesothelioma.

Genetic Associations

Associations between germ-line genetic mutations and peritoneal malignant mesothelioma are limited to rare case reports, and studies of gene polymorphisms associated with mesothelioma have been entirely limited to pleural disease to date. Animal studies have suggested that mice heterozygous for a deleterious mutation in the *NF2* gene demonstrate greater susceptibility to mesothelioma upon intraperitoneal injection of crocidolite, and a single case of human peritoneal malignant mesothelioma in a neurofibromatosis type 2 patient has been reported [160, 161]. A single case of an incidentally found epithelioid peritoneal malignant mesothelioma in a 60-year-old woman with a known germ-line *TP53* mutation has also been reported [162].

BAP1 Syndromic Disease

Wiesner et al. have reported a family affected by autosomal-dominant malignant mesothelioma due to a germ-line *BAP-1* mutation, and identified two family members in two different generations affected by peritoneal malignant mesothelioma [128]. FISH failed to demonstrate loss of the *BAP1* in these patients, but immunohistochemical studies demonstrated loss of BAP1 expression, suggesting other mechanisms of BAP1 downregulation. Pilarski et al. described one probable case of peritoneal malignant mesothelioma associated with a germ-line *BAP1* mutation [131]. Two additional familial cases of well-differentiated papillary mesothelioma with confirmed frameshift mutations in exon 9 of the *BAP1* gene have also been recently described, suggesting similar genetic alterations may contribute to biologically distinct entities [163].

References

1. Travis WD, Brambilla E, Müller-Hermelink HK, Harris CC. World Health Organization classification of tumours (pathology and genetics): tumours of the lung, pleura, thymus and heart. Lyon: IARC; 2004.
2. Robinson BM. Malignant pleural mesothelioma: an epidemiological perspective. Ann Cardiothorac Surg. 2012;1(4):491–6.
3. Wagner JC, Sleggs CA, Marchand P. Diffuse pleural mesothelioma and asbestos exposure in the North Western Cape Province. Br J Ind Med. 1960;17:260–71.
4. World Health Organization. Asbestos: elimination of asbestos-related diseases. 2010. http://www.who.int/mediacentre/factsheets/fs343/en/index.html. Accessed 1 Jan 2014.
5. Driscoll T, Nelson DI, Steenland K, Leigh J, Concha-Barrientos M, Fingerhut M, et al. The global burden of disease due to occupational carcinogens. Am J Ind Med. 2005;48(6):419–31.
6. Delgermaa V, Takahashi K, Park EK, Le GV, Hara T, Sorahan T. Global mesothelioma deaths reported to the World Health Organization between 1994 and 2008. Bull World Health Organ. 2011;89(10):716–24, 724A–C.
7. Park EK, Takahashi K, Hoshuyama T, Cheng TJ, Delgermaa V, Le GV, et al. Global magnitude of reported and unreported mesothelioma. Environ Health Perspect. 2011;119(4):514–8.
8. Marinaccio A, Binazzi A, Marzio DD, Scarselli A, Verardo M, Mirabelli D, et al. Pleural malignant mesothelioma epidemic: incidence, modalities of asbestos exposure and occupations involved from the Italian National Register. Int J Cancer. 2012;130(9):2146–54.
9. Aoe K, Hiraki A, Fujimoto N. The first nationwide survival analysis of Japanese mesothelioma patients from Vital Statistics of Japan. J Clin Oncol. 2012;28:abstracte12007.
10. Safe Work Australia. Mesothelioma in Australia Incidence 1982 to 2009 Mortality 1997 to 2011. 2013. http://www.safeworkaustralia.gov.au/sites/swa/about/publications/pages/mesothelioma-in-australia-incidence-1982-to-2009-mortality-1997-to-2011. Accessed 1 Jan 2014.
11. Cancer Research UK. Mesothelioma statistics. 2012. http://www.cancerresearchuk.org/cancer-info.cancerstats/types/Mesothelioma. Accessed 1 Jan 2014.
12. Park EK, Takahashi K, Jiang Y, Movahed M, Kameda T. Elimination of asbestos use and asbestos-related diseases: an unfinished story. Cancer Sci. 2012;103(10):1751–5.
13. Mesothelioma. SEER Incidence 1975–2009. 2011. http://seer.cancer.gov/csr/1975_2009_pops09/results_merged/sect_17_mesothelioma.pdf. Accessed 1 Jan 2014.
14. Weill H, Hughes JM, Churg AM. Changing trends in US mesothelioma incidence. Occup Environ Med. 2004;61(5):438–41.
15. Spirtas R, Heineman EF, Bernstein L, Beebe GW, Keehn RJ, Stark A, et al. Malignant mesothelioma: attributable risk of asbestos exposure. Occup Environ Med. 1994;51(12):804–11.
16. Armstrong BK, de Klerk NH, Musk AW, Hobbs MS. Mortality in miners and millers of crocidolite in Western Australia. Br J Ind Med. 1988;45(1):5–13.
17. Berman DW, Crump KS. Update of potency factors for asbestos-related lung cancer and mesothelioma. Crit Rev Toxicol. 2008;38(Suppl 1):1–47.
18. Price B. Analysis of current trends in United States mesothelioma incidence. Am J Epidemiol. 1997;145(3):211–8.
19. Acheson ED, Gardner MJ, Pippard EC, Grime LP. Mortality of two groups of women who manufactured gas masks from chrysotile and crocidolite asbestos: a 40-year follow-up. Br J Ind Med. 1982;39(4):344–8.
20. Reid A, Heyworth J, de Klerk NH, Musk B. Cancer incidence among women and girls environmentally and occupationally exposed to blue asbestos at Wittenoom, Western Australia. Int J Cancer. 2008;122(10):2337–44.
21. Luo S, Liu X, Mu S, Tsai SP, Wen CP. Asbestos related diseases from environmental exposure to crocidolite in Da-yao, China. I. Review of exposure and epidemiological data. Occup Environ Med. 2003;60(1):35–41, discussion 41–2.

22. Bayram M, Dongel I, Bakan ND, Yalcin H, Cevit R, Dumortier P, et al. High risk of malignant mesothelioma and pleural plaques in subjects born close to ophiolites. Chest. 2013;143(1):164–71.
23. Senyigit A, Babayigit C, Gokirmak M, Topcu F, Asan E, Coskunsel M, et al. Incidence of malignant pleural mesothelioma due to environmental asbestos fiber exposure in the southeast of Turkey. Respiration. 2000;67(6):610–4.
24. Pan XL, Day HW, Wang W, Beckett LA, Schenker MB. Residential proximity to naturally occurring asbestos and mesothelioma risk in California. Am J Respir Crit Care Med. 2005;172(8):1019–25.
25. van der Bij S, Koffijberg H, Burgers JA, Baas P, van de Vijver MJ, de Mol BA, et al. Prognosis and prognostic factors of patients with mesothelioma: a population-based study. Br J Cancer. 2012;107(1):161–4.
26. Skammeritz E, Omland LH, Johansen JP, Omland O. Asbestos exposure and survival in malignant mesothelioma: a description of 122 consecutive cases at an occupational clinic. Int J Occup Environ Med. 2011;2(4):224–36.
27. Krug LM, Pass HI, Rusch VW, Kindler HL, Sugarbaker DJ, Rosenzweig KE, et al. Multicenter phase II trial of neoadjuvant pemetrexed plus cisplatin followed by extrapleural pneumonectomy and radiation for malignant pleural mesothelioma. J Clin Oncol. 2009;27(18):3007–13.
28. Milano MT, Zhang H. Malignant pleural mesothelioma: a population-based study of survival. J Thorac Oncol. 2010;5(11):1841–8.
29. Flores RM, Zakowski M, Venkatraman E, Krug L, Rosenzweig K, Dycoco J, et al. Prognostic factors in the treatment of malignant pleural mesothelioma at a large tertiary referral center. J Thorac Oncol. 2007;2(10):957–65.
30. Edge S, Byrd D, Compton C, Fritz A, Greene F, Trotti A, editors. AJCC cancer staging manual. 7th ed. New York: Springer; 2010.
31. Pooley FD, Clark N. Fiber dimensions and aspect ratio of crocidolite, chrysotile and amosite particles detected in lung tissue specimens. Ann N Y Acad Sci. 1979;330:711–6.
32. Davis JM, Addison J, Bolton RE, Donaldson K, Jones AD, Smith T. The pathogenicity of long versus short fibre samples of amosite asbestos administered to rats by inhalation and intraperitoneal injection. Br J Exp Pathol. 1986;67(3):415–30.
33. Goodglick LA, Kane AB. Cytotoxicity of long and short crocidolite asbestos fibers in vitro and in vivo. Cancer Res. 1990;50(16):5153–63.
34. Berman DW, Crump KS. A meta-analysis of asbestos-related cancer risk that addresses fiber size and mineral type. Crit Rev Toxicol. 2008;38(Suppl 1):49–73.
35. Donaldson K, Murphy FA, Duffin R, Poland CA. Asbestos, carbon nanotubes and the pleural mesothelium: a review of the hypothesis regarding the role of long fibre retention in the parietal pleura, inflammation and mesothelioma. Part Fibre Toxicol. 2010;7:5–8977, 7–5.
36. Jasani B, Gibbs A. Mesothelioma not associated with asbestos exposure. Arch Pathol Lab Med. 2012;136(3):262–7.
37. Donaldson K. The inhalation toxicology of p-aramid fibrils. Crit Rev Toxicol. 2009;39(6):487–500.
38. Hodgson JT, Darnton A. The quantitative risks of mesothelioma and lung cancer in relation to asbestos exposure. Ann Occup Hyg. 2000;44(8):565–601.
39. Becklake MR. Occupational lung disease–past record and future trend using the asbestos case as an example. Clin Invest Med. 1983;6(4):305–17.
40. Churg A. Analysis of lung asbestos content. Br J Ind Med. 1991;48(10):649–52.
41. Churg AM, Myers JL, Tazelaar HD, Wright JL, editors. Thurlbeck's Pathology of the Lung. 3rd ed. New York: Thieme Medical Publishers; 2005.
42. Pylev LN. Pretumorous lesions and lung and pleural tumours induced by asbestos in rats, Syrian golden hamsters and Macaca mulatta (rhesus) monkeys. IARC Sci Publ. 1980;30(30):343–55.
43. Phillips JI, Murray J. Malignant mesothelioma in a patient with anthophyllite asbestos fibres in the lungs. Ann Occup Hyg. 2010;54(4):412–6.

44. Sullivan PA. Vermiculite, respiratory disease, and asbestos exposure in Libby, Montana: update of a cohort mortality study. Environ Health Perspect. 2007;115(4):579–85.
45. Gylseth B, Norseth T, Skaug V. Amphibole fibers in a taconite mine and in the lungs of the miners. Am J Ind Med. 1981;2(2):175–84.
46. OSHA standards. OSHA standards. 1996. https://www.osha.gov/SLTC/asbestos/standards.html. Accessed 1 Jan 2014.
47. Asbestos Laws and Regulations. Asbestos Laws and Regulations. 2013. http://www2.epa.gov/asbestos/asbestos-laws-and-regulations. Accessed 1 Jan 2014.
48. US Federal Bans on Asbestos. US Federal Bans on Asbestos. 2013. http://www2.epa.gov/asbestos/us-federal-bans-asbestos. Accessed 1 Jan 2014.
49. Finley BL, Pierce JS, Paustenbach DJ, Scott LL, Lievense L, Scott PK, et al. Malignant pleural mesothelioma in US automotive mechanics: reported vs expected number of cases from 1975 to 2007. Regul Toxicol Pharmacol. 2012;64(1):104–16.
50. Lin S, Wang X, Yu IT, Yano E, Courtice M, Qiu H, et al. Cause-specific mortality in relation to chrysotile-asbestos exposure in a Chinese cohort. J Thorac Oncol. 2012;7(7):1109–14.
51. Newman RH. Fine biogenic silica fibres in sugar cane: a possible hazard. Ann Occup Hyg 1986;30(3):365–70.
52. Rothschild H, Mulvey JJ. An increased risk for lung cancer mortality associated with sugarcane farming. J Natl Cancer Inst. 1982;68(5):755–60.
53. Baris I, Simonato L, Artvinli M, Pooley F, Saracci R, Skidmore J, et al. Epidemiological and environmental evidence of the health effects of exposure to erionite fibres: a four-year study in the Cappadocian region of Turkey. Int J Cancer. 1987;39(1):10–7.
54. Peterson JT Jr, Greenberg SD, Buffler PA. Non-asbestos-related malignant mesothelioma. A review. Cancer. 1984;54(5):951–60.
55. Straif K, Benbrahim-Tallaa L, Baan R, Grosse Y, Secretan B, El Ghissassi F, et al. A review of human carcinogens–part C: metals, arsenic, dusts, and fibres. Lancet Oncol. 2009;10(5):453–4.
56. Carbone M, Baris YI, Bertino P, Brass B, Comertpay S, Dogan AU, et al. Erionite exposure in North Dakota and Turkish villages with mesothelioma. Proc Natl Acad Sci USA. 2011;108(33):13618–23.
57. Van Gosen BS, Blitz TA, Plumlee GS, Meeker GP, Pierson MP. Geologic occurrences of erionite in the United States: an emerging national public health concern for respiratory disease. Environ Geochem Health. 2013;35(4):419–30.
58. Kliment CR, Clemens K, Oury TD. North american erionite-associated mesothelioma with pleural plaques and pulmonary fibrosis: a case report. Int J Clin Exp Pathol. 2009;2(4):407–10.
59. Comba P, Gianfagna A, Paoletti L. Pleural mesothelioma cases in Biancavilla are related to a new fluoro-edenite fibrous amphibole. Arch Environ Health. 2003;58(4):229–32.
60. Baan RA, Grosse Y. Man-made mineral (vitreous) fibres: evaluations of cancer hazards by the IARC Monographs Programme. Mutat Res. 2004;553(1–2):43–58.
61. LeMasters GK, Lockey JE, Yiin JH, Hilbert TJ, Levin LS, Rice CH. Mortality of workers occupationally exposed to refractory ceramic fibers. J Occup Environ Med. 2003;45(4):440–50.
62. Lockey JE, LeMasters GK, Levin L, Rice C, Yiin J, Reutman S, et al. A longitudinal study of chest radiographic changes of workers in the refractory ceramic fiber industry. Chest. 2002;121(6):2044–51.
63. Poland CA, Duffin R, Kinloch I, Maynard A, Wallace WA, Seaton A, et al. Carbon nanotubes introduced into the abdominal cavity of mice show asbestos-like pathogenicity in a pilot study. Nat Nanotechnol. 2008;3(7):423–8.
64. Jaurand MC, Renier A, Daubriac J. Mesothelioma: do asbestos and carbon nanotubes pose the same health risk? Part Fibre Toxicol. 2009;6:16–8977, 6–16.
65. Mazzoni E, Corallini A, Cristaudo A, Taronna A, Tassi G, Manfrini M, et al. High prevalence of serum antibodies reacting with simian virus 40 capsid protein mimotopes in patients

affected by malignant pleural mesothelioma. Proc Natl Acad Sci U S A. 2012;109(44):18066–71.
66. Price MJ, Darnton AJ, McElvenny DM, Hodgson JT. Simian virus 40 and mesothelioma in Great Britain. Occup Med (Lond). 2007;57(8):564–8.
67. Cicala C, Pompetti F, Carbone M. SV40 induces mesotheliomas in hamsters. Am J Pathol. 1993;142(5):1524–33.
68. Carbone M, Pass HI, Miele L, Bocchetta M. New developments about the association of SV40 with human mesothelioma. Oncogene. 2003;22(33):5173–80.
69. Carbone M, Pass HI. Evolving aspects of mesothelioma carcinogenesis: SV40 and genetic predisposition. J Thorac Oncol. 2006;1(2):169–71.
70. Carbone M, Pass HI, Rizzo P, Marinetti M, Di Muzio M, Mew DJ, et al. Simian virus 40-like DNA sequences in human pleural mesothelioma. Oncogene. 1994;9(6):1781–90.
71. Cristaudo A, Foddis R, Vivaldi A, Buselli R, Gattini V, Guglielmi G, et al. SV40 enhances the risk of malignant mesothelioma among people exposed to asbestos: a molecular epidemiologic case-control study. Cancer Res. 2005;65(8):3049–52.
72. Gee GV, Stanifer ML, Christensen BC, Atwood WJ, Ugolini D, Bonassi S, et al. SV40 associated miRNAs are not detectable in mesotheliomas. Br J Cancer. 2010;103(6):885–8.
73. Strickler HD, Goedert JJ, Fleming M, Travis WD, Williams AE, Rabkin CS, et al. Simian virus 40 and pleural mesothelioma in humans. Cancer Epidemiol Biomarkers Prev. 1996;5(6):473–5.
74. Ziegler A, Seemayer CA, Hinterberger M, Vogt P, Bigosch C, Gautschi O, et al. Low prevalence of SV40 in Swiss mesothelioma patients after elimination of false-positive PCR results. Lung Cancer. 2007;57(3):282–91.
75. Pepper C, Jasani B, Navabi H, Wynford-Thomas D, Gibbs AR. Simian virus 40 large T antigen (SV40LTAg) primer specific DNA amplification in human pleural mesothelioma tissue. Thorax. 1996;51(11):1074–6.
76. Lopez-Rios F, Illei PB, Rusch V, Ladanyi M. Evidence against a role for SV40 infection in human mesotheliomas and high risk of false-positive PCR results owing to presence of SV40 sequences in common laboratory plasmids. Lancet. 2004;364(9440):1157–66.
77. Rollison DE, Page WF, Crawford H, Gridley G, Wacholder S, Martin J, et al. Case-control study of cancer among US Army veterans exposed to simian virus 40-contaminated adenovirus vaccine. Am J Epidemiol. 2004;160(4):317–24.
78. Engels EA, Katki HA, Nielsen NM, Winther JF, Hjalgrim H, Gjerris F, et al. Cancer incidence in Denmark following exposure to poliovirus vaccine contaminated with simian virus 40. J Natl Cancer Inst. 2003;95(7):532–9.
79. Strickler HD, Rosenberg PS, Devesa SS, Hertel J, Fraumeni JF, Jr, Goedert JJ. Contamination of poliovirus vaccines with simian virus 40 (1955–1963) and subsequent cancer rates. JAMA. 1998;279(4):292–5.
80. Anderson KA, Hurley WC, Hurley BT, Ohrt DW. Malignant pleural mesothelioma following radiotherapy in a 16-year-old boy. Cancer. 1985;56(2):273–6.
81. Antman KH, Corson JM, Li FP, Greenberger J, Sytkowski A, Henson DE, et al. Malignant mesothelioma following radiation exposure. J Clin Oncol. 1983;1(11):695–700.
82. Cavazza A, Travis LB, Travis WD, Wolfe JT 3rd, Foo ML, Gillespie DJ, et al. Post-irradiation malignant mesothelioma. Cancer. 1996;77(7):1379–85.
83. Gilks B, Hegedus C, Freeman H, Fratkin L, Churg A. Malignant peritoneal mesothelioma after remote abdominal radiation. Cancer. 1988;61(10):2019–21.
84. Hofmann J, Mintzer D, Warhol MJ. Malignant mesothelioma following radiation therapy. Am J Med. 1994;97(4):379–82.
85. Lerman Y, Learman Y, Schachter P, Herceg E, Lieberman Y, Yellin A. Radiation associated malignant pleural mesothelioma. Thorax. 1991;46(6):463–4.
86. Pappo AS, Santana VM, Furman WL, Kun LE, Walter AW, Jenkins JJ, et al. Post-irradiation malignant mesothelioma. Cancer. 1997;79(1):192–3.
87. Stock RJ, Fu YS, Carter JR. Malignant peritoneal mesothelioma following radiotherapy for seminoma of the testis. Cancer. 1979;44(3):914–9.

88. Weissmann LB, Corson JM, Neugut AI, Antman KH. Malignant mesothelioma following treatment for Hodgkin's disease. J Clin Oncol. 1996;14(7):2098–100.
89. Witherby SM, Butnor KJ, Grunberg SM. Malignant mesothelioma following thoracic radiotherapy for lung cancer. Lung Cancer. 2007;57(3):410–3.
90. Shannon VR, Nesbitt JC, Libshitz HI. Malignant pleural mesothelioma after radiation therapy for breast cancer. A report of two additional patients. Cancer. 1995;76(3):437–41.
91. Brown LM, Howard RA, Travis LB. The risk of secondary malignancies over 30 years after the treatment of non-Hodgkin lymphoma. Cancer. 2006;107(11):2741–2; author reply 2742.
92. De Bruin ML, Burgers JA, Baas P, van Veer MB, Noordijk EM, Louwman MW, et al. Malignant mesothelioma after radiation treatment for Hodgkin lymphoma. Blood. 2009;113(16):3679–81.
93. Deutsch M, Land SR, Begovic M, Cecchini R, Wolmark N. An association between postoperative radiotherapy for primary breast cancer in 11 National Surgical Adjuvant Breast and Bowel Project (NSABP) studies and the subsequent appearance of pleural mesothelioma. Am J Clin Oncol. 2007;30(3):294–6.
94. Hodgson DC, Gilbert ES, Dores GM, Schonfeld SJ, Lynch CF, Storm H, et al. Long-term solid cancer risk among 5-year survivors of Hodgkin's lymphoma. J Clin Oncol. 2007;25(12):1489–97.
95. Neugut AI, Ahsan H, Antman KH. Incidence of malignant pleural mesothelioma after thoracic radiotherapy. Cancer. 1997;80(5):948–50.
96. Teta MJ, Lau E, Sceurman BK, Wagner ME. Therapeutic radiation for lymphoma: risk of malignant mesothelioma. Cancer. 2007;109(7):1432–8.
97. Tward JD, Wendland MM, Shrieve DC, Szabo A, Gaffney DK. The risk of secondary malignancies over 30 years after the treatment of non-Hodgkin lymphoma. Cancer. 2006;107(1):108–15.
98. Dahlgren S. Effects of locally deposited colloidal thorium dioxide. Ann NY Acad Sci. 1967;145(3):786–90.
99. Goodman JE, Nascarella MA, Valberg PA. Ionizing radiation: a risk factor for mesothelioma. Cancer Causes Control 2009;20(8):1237–54.
100. Mizuki M, Yukishige K, Abe Y, Tsuda T. A case of malignant pleural mesothelioma following exposure to atomic radiation in Nagasaki. Respirology. 1997;2(3):201–5.
101. Vianna NJ, Polan AK. Non-occupational exposure to asbestos and malignant mesothelioma in females. Lancet. 1978;1(8073):1061–3.
102. Risberg B, Nickels J, Wagermark J. Familial clustering of malignant mesothelioma. Cancer. 1980;45(9):2422–7.
103. Ascoli V, Cavone D, Merler E, Barbieri PG, Romeo L, Nardi F, et al. Mesothelioma in blood related subjects: report of 11 clusters among 1954 Italy cases and review of the literature. Am J Ind Med. 2007;50(5):357–69.
104. Dawson A, Gibbs A, Browne K, Pooley F, Griffiths M. Familial mesothelioma. Details of 17 cases with histopathologic findings and mineral analysis. Cancer. 1992;70(5):1183–7.
105. Hammar SP, Bockus D, Remington F, Freidman S, LaZerte G. Familial mesothelioma: a report of two families. Hum Pathol. 1989;20(2):107–12.
106. Lynch HT, Katz D, Markvicka SE. Familial mesothelioma: review and family study. Cancer Genet Cytogenet. 1985;15(1–2):25–35.
107. Landi S, Gemignani F, Neri M, Barale R, Bonassi S, Bottari F, et al. Polymorphisms of glutathione-S-transferase M1 and manganese superoxide dismutase are associated with the risk of malignant pleural mesothelioma. Int J Cancer. 2007;120(12):2739–43.
108. de Klerk N, Alfonso H, Olsen N, Reid A, Sleith J, Palmer L, et al. Familial aggregation of malignant mesothelioma in former workers and residents of Wittenoom, Western Australia. Int J Cancer. 2013;132(6):1423–8.
109. Bianchi C, Brollo A, Ramani L, Bianchi T, Giarelli L. Familial mesothelioma of the pleura–a report of 40 cases. Ind Health. 2004;42(2):235–9.

110. Roushdy-Hammady I, Siegel J, Emri S, Testa JR, Carbone M. Genetic-susceptibility factor and malignant mesothelioma in the Cappadocian region of Turkey. Lancet. 2001;357(9254):444–5.
111. Saracci R, Simonato L. Familial malignant mesothelioma. Lancet. 2001;358(9295):1813–4.
112. Dogan AU, Baris YI, Dogan M, Emri S, Steele I, Elmishad AG, et al. Genetic predisposition to fiber carcinogenesis causes a mesothelioma epidemic in Turkey. Cancer Res. 2006;66(10):5063–8.
113. Carbone M, Emri S, Dogan AU, Steele I, Tuncer M, Pass HI, et al. A mesothelioma epidemic in Cappadocia: scientific developments and unexpected social outcomes. Nat Rev Cancer. 2007;7(2):147–54.
114. Metintas M, Hillerdal G, Metintas S, Dumortier P. Endemic malignant mesothelioma: exposure to erionite is more important than genetic factors. Arch Environ Occup Health. 2010;65(2):86–93.
115. Huncharek M. Genetic factors in the aetiology of malignant mesothelioma. Eur J Cancer. 1995;31A(11):1741–7.
116. Neri M, Ugolini D, Dianzani I, Gemignani F, Landi S, Cesario A, et al. Genetic susceptibility to malignant pleural mesothelioma and other asbestos-associated diseases. Mutat Res. 2008;659(1–2):126–36.
117. Fleury-Feith J, Lecomte C, Renier A, Matrat M, Kheuang L, Abramowski V, et al. Hemizygosity of Nf2 is associated with increased susceptibility to asbestos-induced peritoneal tumours. Oncogene. 2003;22(24):3799–805.
118. Cadby G, Mukherjee S, Musk AW, Reid A, Garlepp M, Dick I, et al. A genome-wide association study for malignant mesothelioma risk. Lung Cancer. 2013;82(1):1–8.
119. Baser ME, Rai H, Wallace AJ, Evans DG. Neurofibromatosis 2 (NF2) and malignant mesothelioma in a man with a constitutional NF2 missense mutation. Fam Cancer. 2005;4(4):321–2.
120. Hirvonen A, Pelin K, Tammilehto L, Karjalainen A, Mattson K, Linnainmaa K. Inherited GSTM1 and NAT2 defects as concurrent risk modifiers in asbestos-related human malignant mesothelioma. Cancer Res. 1995;55(14):2981–3.
121. Gemignani F, Neri M, Bottari F, Barale R, Canessa PA, Canzian F, et al. Risk of malignant pleural mesothelioma and polymorphisms in genes involved in the genome stability and xenobiotics metabolism. Mutat Res. 2009;671(1–2):76–83.
122. Betti M, Ferrante D, Padoan M, Guarrera S, Giordano M, Aspesi A, et al. XRCC1 and ERCC1 variants modify malignant mesothelioma risk: a case-control study. Mutat Res. 2011;708(1–2):11–20.
123. Matullo G, Guarrera S, Betti M, Fiorito G, Ferrante D, Voglino F, et al. Genetic variants associated with increased risk of malignant pleural mesothelioma: a genome-wide association study. PLoS One. 2013;8(4):e61253.
124. Testa JR, Cheung M, Pei J, Below JE, Tan Y, Sementino E, et al. Germline BAP1 mutations predispose to malignant mesothelioma. Nat Genet. 2011;43(10):1022–5.
125. Bott M, Brevet M, Taylor BS, Shimizu S, Ito T, Wang L, et al. The nuclear deubiquitinase BAP1 is commonly inactivated by somatic mutations and 3p21.1 losses in malignant pleural mesothelioma. Nat Genet. 2011;43(7):668–72.
126. Yoshikawa Y, Sato A, Tsujimura T, Emi M, Morinaga T, Fukuoka K, et al. Frequent inactivation of the BAP1 gene in epithelioid-type malignant mesothelioma. Cancer Sci. 2012;103(5):868–74.
127. Zauderer MG, Bott M, McMillan R, Sima CS, Rusch V, Krug LM, et al. Clinical characteristics of patients with malignant pleural mesothelioma harboring somatic BAP1 mutations. J Thorac Oncol. 2013;8(11):1430–3.
128. Wiesner T, Fried I, Ulz P, Stacher E, Popper H, Murali R, et al. Toward an improved definition of the tumor spectrum associated with BAP1 germline mutations. J Clin Oncol. 2012;30(32):e337–40.

129. Carbone M, Ferris LK, Baumann F, Napolitano A, Lum CA, Flores EG, et al. BAP1 cancer syndrome: malignant mesothelioma, uveal and cutaneous melanoma, and MBAITs. J Transl Med. 2012;10:179–5876, 10–179.
130. Popova T, Hebert L, Jacquemin V, Gad S, Caux-Moncoutier V, Dubois-d'Enghien C, et al. Germline BAP1 mutations predispose to renal cell carcinomas. Am J Hum Genet. 2013;92(6):974–80.
131. Pilarski R, Cebulla CM, Massengill JB, Rai K, Rich T, Strong L, et al. Expanding the clinical phenotype of hereditary BAP1 cancer predisposition syndrome, reporting three new cases. Genes Chromosomes Cancer. 2014;53(2):177–82.
132. Plaus WJ. Peritoneal mesothelioma. Arch Surg. 1988;123(6):763–6.
133. Kannerstein M, Churg J. Peritoneal mesothelioma. Hum Pathol. 1977;8(1):83–94.
134. Baker PM, Clement PB, Young RH. Malignant peritoneal mesothelioma in women: a study of 75 cases with emphasis on their morphologic spectrum and differential diagnosis. Am J Clin Pathol. 2005;123(5):724–37.
135. Daya D, McCaughey WT. Well-differentiated papillary mesothelioma of the peritoneum. A clinicopathologic study of 22 cases. Cancer. 1990;65(2):292–6.
136. Malpica A, Sant'Ambrogio S, Deavers MT, Silva EG. Well-differentiated papillary mesothelioma of the female peritoneum: a clinicopathologic study of 26 cases. Am J Surg Pathol. 2012;36(1):117–27.
137. Sawh RN, Malpica A, Deavers MT, Liu J, Silva EG. Benign cystic mesothelioma of the peritoneum: a clinicopathologic study of 17 cases and immunohistochemical analysis of estrogen and progesterone receptor status. Hum Pathol. 2003;34(4):369–74.
138. Weiss SW, Tavassoli FA. Multicystic mesothelioma. An analysis of pathologic findings and biologic behavior in 37 cases. Am J Surg Pathol. 1988;12(10):737–46.
139. Manzini Vde P, Recchia L, Cafferata M, Porta C, Siena S, Giannetta L, et al. Malignant peritoneal mesothelioma: a multicenter study on 81 cases. Ann Oncol. 2010;21(2):348–53.
140. Boffetta P. Epidemiology of peritoneal mesothelioma: a review. Ann Oncol. 2007;18(6):985–90.
141. Kindler HL. Peritoneal mesothelioma: the site of origin matters. Am Soc Clin Oncol Educ Book. 2013:182–8.
142. Teta MJ, Mink PJ, Lau E, Sceurman BK, Foster ED. US mesothelioma patterns 1973–2002: indicators of change and insights into background rates. Eur J Cancer Prev. 2008;17(6):525–34.
143. Mirabelli D, Roberti S, Gangemi M, Rosato R, Ricceri F, Merler E, et al. Survival of peritoneal malignant mesothelioma in Italy: a population-based study. Int J Cancer. 2009;124(1):194–200.
144. Spirtas R, Heineman EF, Bernstein L, Beebe GW, Keehn RJ, Stark A, et al. Malignant mesothelioma: attributable risk of asbestos exposure. Occup Environ Med. 1994;51(12):804–11.
145. Cocco P, Dosemeci M. Peritoneal cancer and occupational exposure to asbestos: results from the application of a job-exposure matrix. Am J Ind Med. 1999;35(1):9–14.
146. Coggon D, Inskip H, Winter P, Pannett B. Differences in occupational mortality from pleural cancer, peritoneal cancer, and asbestosis. Occup Environ Med. 1995;52(11):775–7.
147. Cao C, Yan TD, Deraco M, Elias D, Glehen O, Levine EA, et al. Importance of gender in diffuse malignant peritoneal mesothelioma. Ann Oncol. 2012;23(6):1494–8.
148. Yan TD, Popa E, Brun EA, Cerruto CA, Sugarbaker PH. Sex difference in diffuse malignant peritoneal mesothelioma. Br J Surg. 2006;93(12):1536–42.
149. CDC Malignant Mesothelioma Mortality–United States, 1999–2005. CDC Malignant Mesothelioma Mortality–United States, 1999–2005. 2009. http://www.cdc.gov/mmwr/preview/mmwrhtml/mm5815a3.htm. 2014.
150. Ozesmi M, Patiroglu TE, Hillerdal G, Ozesmi C. Peritoneal mesothelioma and malignant lymphoma in mice caused by fibrous zeolite. Br J Ind Med. 1985;42(11):746–9.
151. Baris YI, Grandjean P. Prospective study of mesothelioma mortality in Turkish villages with exposure to fibrous zeolite. J Natl Cancer Inst. 2006;98(6):414–7.

152. Varga C, Szendi K. Carbon nanotubes induce granulomas but not mesotheliomas. In Vivo. 2010;24(2):153–6.
153. Shivapurkar N, Wiethege T, Wistuba II, Milchgrub S, Muller KM, Gazdar AF. Presence of simian virus 40 sequences in malignant pleural, peritoneal and noninvasive mesotheliomas. Int J Cancer. 20001;85(5):743–5.
154. Maurer R, Egloff B. Malignant peritoneal mesothelioma after cholangiography with thorotrast. Cancer. 1975;36(4):1381–5.
155. Andersson M, Carstensen B, Storm HH. Mortality and cancer incidence after cerebral arteriography with or without Thorotrast. Radiat Res. 1995;142(3):305–20.
156. van Kaick G, Dalheimer A, Hornik S, Kaul A, Liebermann D, Luhrs H, et al. The german thorotrast study: recent results and assessment of risks. Radiat Res. 1999;152(6 Suppl):S64–71.
157. Ugolini D, Neri M, Ceppi M, Cesario A, Dianzani I, Filiberti R, et al. Genetic susceptibility to malignant mesothelioma and exposure to asbestos: the influence of the familial factor. Mutat Res. 2008;658(3):162–71.
158. Tangjitgamol S, Erlichman J, Northrup H, Malpica A, Wang X, Lee E, et al. Benign multicystic peritoneal mesothelioma: cases reports in the family with diverticulosis and literature review. Int J Gynecol Cancer. 2005;15(6):1101–7.
159. Picklesimer AH, Zanagnolo V, Niemann TH, Eaton LA, Copeland LJ. Case report: malignant peritoneal mesothelioma in two siblings. Gynecol Oncol. 2005;99(2):512–6.
160. Baser ME, De Rienzo A, Altomare D, Balsara BR, Hedrick NM, Gutmann DH, et al. Neurofibromatosis 2 and malignant mesothelioma. Neurology. 2002;59(2):290–1.
161. Fleury-Feith J, Lecomte C, Renier A, Matrat M, Kheuang L, Abramowski V, et al. Hemizygosity of Nf2 is associated with increased susceptibility to asbestos-induced peritoneal tumours. Oncogene. 2003;22(24):3799–805.
162. Ceelen WP, Van Dalen T, Van Bockstal M, Libbrecht L, Sijmons RH. Malignant peritoneal mesothelioma in a patient with Li-Fraumeni syndrome. J Clin Oncol. 2011;29(17):e503–5.
163. Ribeiro C, Campelos S, Moura CS, Machado JC, Justino A, Parente B. Well-differentiated papillary mesothelioma: clustering in a Portuguese family with a germline BAP1 mutation. Ann Oncol. 2013;24(8):2147–50.

Chapter 3
Clinical and Radiologic Features

Anja C. Roden and Christine U. Lee

Introduction

Patients with diffuse malignant pleural mesothelioma often have an insidious onset of symptoms. Nonspecific symptoms may be present for several months and even years until a diagnosis is rendered. At that time, many of the symptoms reflect advanced disease with signs of progressive local expansion of the tumor, tumor invasion into surrounding structures, and/or tumor spread. A combination of patient symptoms and signs at the time of diagnosis is common (Table 3.1). The two most common symptoms are dyspnea and chest pain which are reported in approximately 90% of patients [1].

Diffuse Malignant Pleural Mesothelioma: Clinical Signs and Symptoms

Dyspnea

The most common cause of dyspnea in patients with diffuse malignant pleural mesothelioma is a large pleural effusion [2]. Pleural effusion in diffuse malignant pleural mesothelioma is usually unilateral, present at the site of disease. The effusion might cause atelectasis and/or pneumonia of the underlying lung and might restrict

---

A. C. Roden (✉)
Department of Laboratory Medicine and Pathology, Mayo Clinic,
200 First Street SW, Rochester, MN 55905, USA
e-mail: Roden.anja@mayo.edu

C. U. Lee
Department of Radiology, Mayo Clinic, 200 First Street SW, Rochester, MN, USA

© Springer Science+Business Media New York 2015
T. C. Allen (ed.), *Diffuse Malignant Mesothelioma,* DOI 10.1007/978-1-4939-2374-8_3

Table 3.1 Signs and symptoms of patients with diffuse malignant pleural mesothelioma

Signs and symptoms	Percent patients
Pulmonary	
Dyspnea [1, 7, 23, 24, 31, 47]	35–82
Pleural effusion [6, 7, 31, 85]	54–87
Chest pain [1, 7, 23, 24, 31, 47, 85]	35–71
Cough [7, 23, 31, 47]	6–37
Increased sputum production [31]	18
Pneumothorax/hydropneumothorax [6, 85]	≤10
Interstitial lung disease [9–13]	≤6
Systemic	
Fatigue [7,31]	18–33
Weight loss [7, 24, 31, 47, 85]	9–59
Anorexia [7]	11
Fever, chills, or sweat [7, 23, 47, 85]	6–33
Pericardial effusions [47]	9
Sensation of heaviness or fullness of chest [7]	7
Hoarseness, early satiety, myalgia [7]	≤3 each
No symptoms, incidental diagnosis [23, 31, 47]	3–8

the movement of the ipsilateral hemidiaphragm. In advanced disease, malignant mesothelioma usually encases the lung resulting in restrictive lung function and/or pneumonia [3].

Patients might present with pneumothorax or hydropneumothorax which usually also results in dyspnea (Fig. 3.1). Once thought to be rare, pneumothorax or hydropneumothorax as initial presentation is now understood to occur in up to 10% of cases. In a series of 91 patients who underwent pleurectomy for spontaneous pneumothorax, five patients (4.3%) were diagnosed with malignant mesothelioma [4]. Alkhuja et al. described four patients who presented with spontaneous pneumothorax and were ultimately diagnosed with malignant mesothelioma [5]. Two of the four patients were diagnosed with malignant mesothelioma 12 and 22 months after the initial pneumothorax. Pneumothorax might be under-recognized in this patient population given a recent radiologic study of 92 patients who were diagnosed with malignant pleural mesothelioma between 1997 and 2006 [6]. Nine (of 92) patients (10%) were found to have pneumothorax on computed tomography (CT) imaging studies.

Dyspnea due to mesothelioma might be compounded by other lung diseases that are often present in this patient population such as chronic obstructive pulmonary disease, asbestosis, or ischemic heart disease [3].

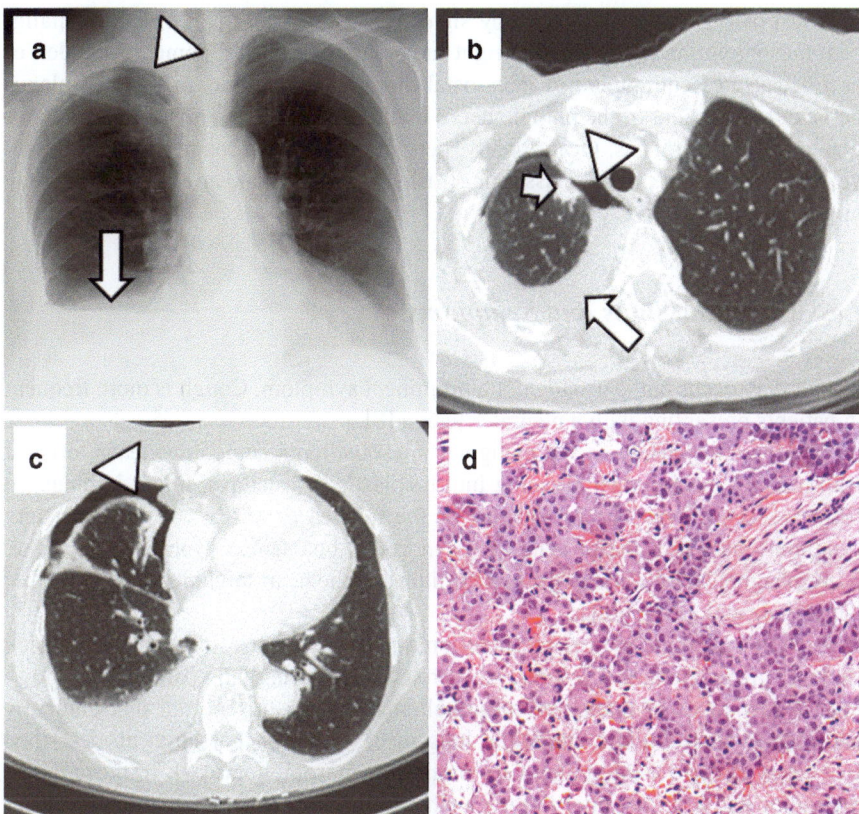

Fig. 3.1 This 80-year-old woman noted increasing exertional dyspnea over the past month along with dry cough. A chest X-ray revealed right-sided pleural fluid (*arrow*) and a small pneumothorax (*arrowhead*; hydropneumothorax) (**a**). A subsequent CT scan confirmed these findings (right-sided pleural effusion, *long arrow*; pneumothorax, *arrowhead*) and also revealed a 1.3 cm nodule in the right apex (*short arrow*), moderate volume loss of the right middle and lower lobes and thickening of the visceral pleura (**b, c**). The left lung and abdomen appear unremarkable. Biopsy from the right visceral pleura confirmed malignant mesothelioma, epithelioid type (**d**). *CT* computed tomography

Chest Pain

Chest pain in malignant pleural mesothelioma is most often of nonpleuritic quality, although pleuritic chest pain can also occur. In contrast to the nonpleuritic chest pain, pleuritic pain is typically characterized by a sudden, intense, and sometimes stabbing or shooting chest pain that is usually most severe when the lungs move during breathing, coughing, sneezing, or even talking. In a study by Adams et al., 62 patients (69 %) presented with chest pain; in 56 patients the chest pain was of nonpleuritic quality and only six patients had pleuritic chest pain [7].

Chest pain is generally caused by significant chest wall invasion by the malignant mesothelioma [2]. The pain might radiate to the upper abdomen, shoulder, or arm because of entrapment of intercostal thoracic, autonomic, or brachial plexus nerves. Involvement of the phrenic nerve by the mesothelioma might lead to hemidiaphragmatic paralysis. Occasionally, persistent chest wall pain precedes the development of either pleural masses or effusion by months and an initial chest X-ray might even be negative.

Less Common Signs and Symptoms

Cough may occur but is usually not a prominent symptom. Cough is more frequent in patients presenting with a pleural effusion [8].

The local expansion of the malignant mesothelioma sometimes leads to chest wall masses which, when invading into mediastinal structures, might impinge on large vessels, nerves, the esophagus, or the trachea or airways resulting in rare symptoms such as superior vena cava syndrome, hoarseness, Horner's syndrome, or dysphagia [3]. Invasion of the pericardium and the heart might lead to pericardial tamponade and arrhythmias.

Diffuse malignant pleural mesothelioma typically encases the lungs as a thick rind and grows along the fissures, while relatively sparing lung parenchyma; however, a few cases of malignant mesothelioma have been reported that clinically and radiologically mimic interstitial lung disease [9–13]. Larsen et al. described five cases of diffuse intrapulmonary malignant mesothelioma [9]. In those cases, the tumor had a preferential intraparenchymal growth pattern without significant pleural involvement. All five patients were men with a median age of 56 years. Patients presented with chronic dyspnea, cough, and acute dyspnea with bilateral pneumothorax, and were initially diagnosed as interstitial lung disease based on clinical and radiologic findings. Microscopic pleural involvement was identified in four cases. The median survival of three of the five patients treated with chemotherapy was 28 months [9]. Two patients received no therapy and survived 3 and 4 weeks, respectively.

Diffuse malignant pleural mesothelioma might spread to the abdomen and patients might present with ascites, constipation, or even bowel obstruction. Mesothelioma can also spread to the contralateral hemithorax resulting in bilateral pleural effusion [3].

In rare cases, malignant mesothelioma has been diagnosed at a prior incision site. Guenday et al. reported a 37-year-old woman who underwent pericardiocentesis for pericardial effusion with negative cytologic examination [14]. Seven months later, she presented with a skin lesion at the prior incision site which was found to be malignant mesothelioma. She was also diagnosed with pericardial malignant mesothelioma.

Lymphatic and hematogenous dissemination occurs late in the course of malignant pleural mesothelioma, and is identified fairly commonly in autopsy series. All organs can be involved. Metastatic disease has been described in liver, lung, heart, brain, meninges, thyroid, adrenal glands, kidneys, pancreas, bone, soft tissue, skin, and lymph nodes [15, 16]. Systemic lymphadenopathy is an exceedingly rare initial presentation of malignant mesothelioma with only a few cases being reported. In some of these case reports, the malignant mesothelioma was initially diagnosed in a lymph node, most commonly cervical, supraclavicular, or axillary, which initiated a search for the primary tumor, with peritoneal, pleural, or pericardial mesothelioma subsequently identified [17–21]. In one case of metastatic disease to the neck, the malignant pleural mesothelioma was not identified until 8 months after the initial diagnosis in the lymph node [22].

Other rare presentations include aphonia and dysphagia, abdominal distension, pressure sensation in the abdominal right upper quadrant, nausea, bad taste in the mouth, perceived tachycardia, headache, paraneoplastic syndrome, chest wall lump, lymphadenopathy, and hemoptysis [7, 23].

Time Interval Between Symptoms and Diagnosis

The average time interval between onset of symptoms and diagnosis is usually 2–3 months [3], but insidious and nonspecific symptoms may delay diagnosis up to 3–6 months or more [2, 24]. However, symptoms may present for an even longer time until a diagnosis is established, leading in some cases to long latency periods [5].

Location

Diffuse malignant pleural mesothelioma is slightly more common in the right pleura, and bilateral involvement at initial diagnosis is uncommon. A study by Adams found that the tumor was right sided in 55% of patients, left sided in 41%, and bilateral in 3% [7]. Similarly, in the radiologic study by Seely, the right hemithorax was more commonly involved than the left (61 vs. 36%, respectively), and 3% of patients had bilateral involvement [6]. Tanrikulu et al. studied 363 patients with pleural mesothelioma and also showed that the majority of mesotheliomas were right sided (61%), with only 7% bilateral [24]. In a study of 272 patients with malignant mesothelioma in southeast England, right-sided disease were 1.6 times more common than left-sided disease based on clinical, radiologic, and autopsy data [25].

Table 3.2 Signs and symptoms of patients with diffuse malignant peritoneal mesothelioma

Signs and symptoms	Percent patients
Abdominal	
Abdominal distension/increasing abdominal girth [26, 30, 31]	30–80
Ascites [29, 31, 36]	36–90
Abdominal mass [31, 36]	11–30
Pain [30, 31, 36]	27–69
Hernia [30, 31]	7–12
Diarrhea [36]	17
Vomiting [36]	15
Nausea [31]	11
Bowel obstruction [31]	3
Systemic	
Fatigue [31, 36]	11–43
Weight loss [31, 36]	32–38
Anorexia [31, 36]	27–30
Fever [36]	22
No symptoms, incidental diagnosis [30, 35]	8–17

Diffuse Malignant Peritoneal Mesothelioma: Clinical Signs and Symptoms

There are no signs or symptoms that are specific for diffuse malignant peritoneal mesothelioma (Table 3.2). Due to the nonspecific nature of the presenting symptoms, many patients have already an advanced stage of the disease at the time of diagnosis. Radiological features of peritoneal malignant mesothelioma are also nonspecific and can include ascites and peritoneal thickening, nodularity, or masses with or without omental involvement. Differential considerations include peritoneal carcinomatosis, pseudomyxoma peritonei, peritonitis, cystic lymphangioma, and ovarian neoplasms.

Abdominal Distension

Abdominal distension and/or increasing abdominal girth is the most frequent initial symptom, occurring in 30–80 % of patients with peritoneal malignant mesothelioma [26–28]. It is usually due to ascites or may be due to tumor mass expansion within the abdominal cavity. Ascites is the most common sign, occurring in 90 % of the patients [29]. In contrast to patients with abdominal distension due to excess caloric intake or benign ascites associated with nonmalignant conditions (e.g., cirrhosis) where patients can gain weight, patients with mesothelioma often exhibit weight loss.

Pain

Pain is the second most common symptom in patients with diffuse malignant peritoneal mesothelioma, although in some studies, it was more common than abdominal distension [30, 31] (Fig. 3.2). In most cases, the pain is diffuse and nonspecific, although rarely, patients can present with an acute abdomen secondary to perforation or bowel obstruction [32].

Other Signs and Symptoms

Early satiety, dysphagia, and shortness of breath are other nonspecific symptoms that may occur in patients with peritoneal mesothelioma. These symptoms are likely due to ascites or an enlarging abdominal mass and they can contribute to weight loss, impaired performance status, and fatigue. Abdominal distension may manifest as a new or worsening abdominal wall hernia.

Gastrointestinal complications such as bowel obstruction are usually a manifestation of advanced disease and occur late in the course of the disease [26, 33]. A palpable abdominal mass, deep vein thrombosis, and arterial occlusion may also occur [26, 27].

Malignant peritoneal mesotheliomas of the abdominal cavity can occasionally clinically mimic ovarian tumors, especially in young women. Although malignant peritoneal mesothelioma can secondarily involve the ovaries, patients with malignant peritoneal mesothelioma characteristically present with abdominal disease rather than with ovarian masses. Mani et al. described seven cases of peritoneal mesothelioma in which the initial manifestation was an ovarian mass [34]. The patients, ranging from 22 to 52 years old, underwent surgery with a primary diagnosis of ovarian cancer, exhibiting masses measuring 3.8–9 cm. Four of the seven cases were predominantly cystic and three were solid tumors. Histologically, the cystic tumors were multicystic mesotheliomas, and the three solid tumors were diffuse malignant mesotheliomas.

Occasionally, malignant mesothelioma is an incidental finding during infertility surgery or other gynecologic surgery [30]. In a study of 75 women with malignant peritoneal mesothelioma, 13 (17%) were incidental surgical findings [35].

Time Interval Between Symptoms and Diagnosis

Similar to diffuse malignant pleural mesothelioma, the mean time interval between the onset of symptoms and the establishment of the diagnosis is typically 2–3 months. Manzini et al. found that the median diagnosis time (first symptoms to diagnosis) was 2 months (range, 0–29 months) [36]. Acherman et al. reported a mean

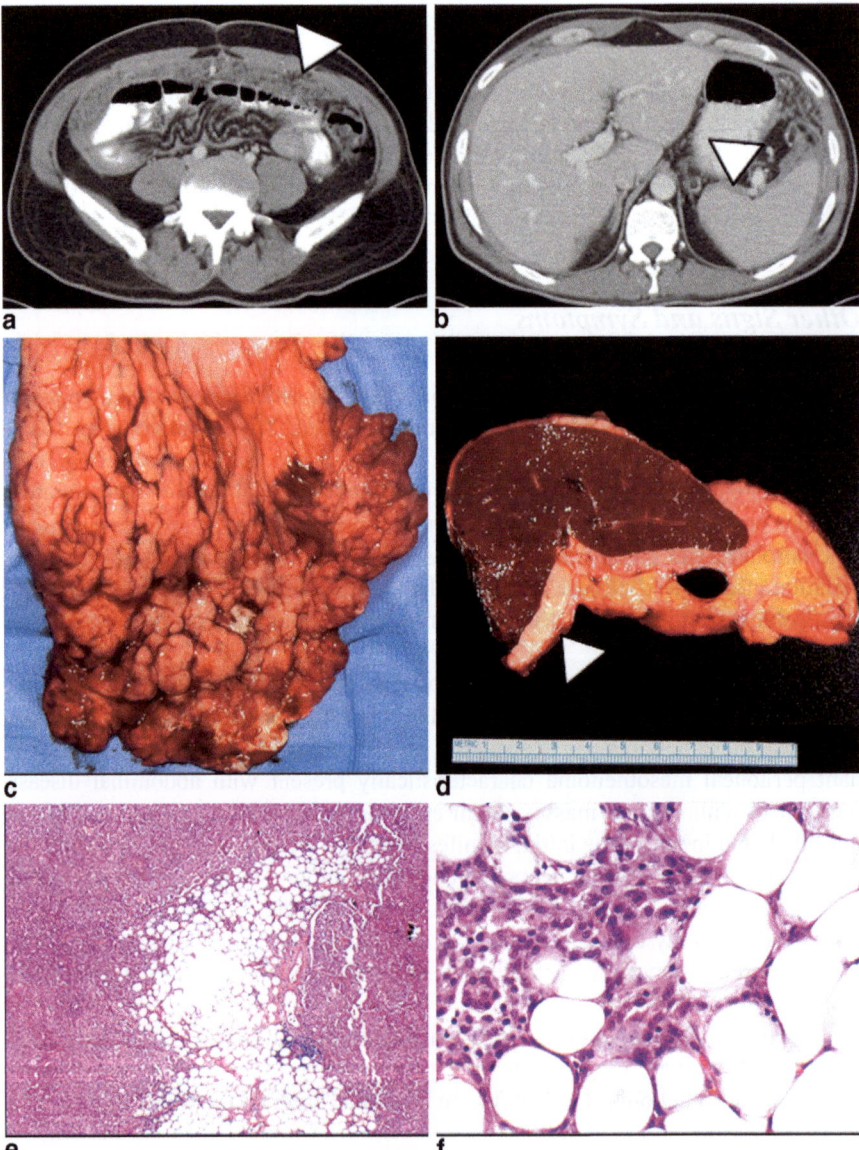

Fig. 3.2 This 48-year-old man presented with abdominal pain, some weight loss over several months, and fatigue. Work-up revealed anemia and a negative colonoscopy. His abdominal symptoms continued and about 2 weeks later, he presented to the emergency department. A CT scan of the abdomen showed diffuse thickening of the omentum (**a**, *arrowhead*) and peritoneal thickening surrounding the spleen (**b**, *arrowhead*). The chest appeared uninvolved. The patient underwent exploratory laparotomy. The omentum was diffusely involved by malignant mesothelioma forming a 38.0 cm mass (**c**) which was resected. The spleen was encased by malignant mesothelioma (**d**, *arrowhead*) and removed. An appendectomy and peritoneal stripping were also performed. Histologic examination, on low power view, shows sheets of epithelioid cells invading into adipose

diagnosis time of 10 months [30]. However, in a few patients, the time between symptoms and diagnosis has been reported in years, reflecting the lack of specific symptoms, the rarity of the disease, and the difficulty in distinguishing between diffuse malignant peritoneal mesothelioma and other primary or metastatic peritoneal tumors [26, 29]. In a study of 75 women with malignant peritoneal mesothelioma, Baker et al. identified four cases with delayed diagnosis between 2 months and 3 years [35]. In these four cases, a diagnosis of florid reactive or atypical mesothelial hyperplasia was made at initial surgery; however, later laparotomy for persistent symptoms showed malignant mesothelioma.

Clinical Presentations Common to Both Diffuse Pleural and Peritoneal Mesothelioma

Paraneoplastic Syndromes

Malignant mesothelioma can be associated with various paraneoplastic syndromes, including thrombocytosis [36], migratory thrombophlebitis, disseminated intravascular coagulation, venous thrombosis [37, 38], thrombotic thrombocytopenic purpura (TTP) [39], Coombs-positive hemolytic anemia, hypoglycemia [27], fever, paraneoplastic hepatopathy [27], sensory–motor polyneuropathy [40], Anti-Ma2 antibody-associated paraneoplastic syndrome (presenting with opsoclonus and diffuse cerebellar signs) [41], anti-Yo-related paraneoplastic cerebellar degeneration [42], renal disease, and hypercalcemia. These paraneoplastic syndromes are of course not unique to malignant mesothelioma and also have been described in other malignancies. Paraneoplastic syndromes are generally seen in the context of advanced disease; however, in some cases, malignant mesothelioma is diagnosed during the workup of the paraneoplastic syndrome. Archer et al. reported a sarcomatoid mesothelioma patient with opsoclonus and diffuse cerebellar signs who had an anti-Ma2 antibody-associated paraneoplastic syndrome [41]. Socola et al. reported a patient who presented with recurrent, rapidly relapsing episodes of thrombotic thrombocytopenic purpura associated with severe abdominal pain culminating in an acute abdomen who was found to have diffuse malignant peritoneal mesothelioma with tumor located in the left side of the pelvis encasing the distal sigmoid colon [39]. Banayan et al. reported a case of a 45-year-old woman with recurrent

---

tissue (**e**). High power view confirms large atypical epithelioid cells with prominent nucleoli. Immunostains performed on a previous biopsy showed that the neoplastic cells are positive for CK7, calretinin, CK5/6, and WT-1, and negative for CK20, synaptophysin, and chromogranin (not shown). The morphologic and immunophenotypic features are consistent with malignant mesothelioma, epithelioid type (**f**), (Magnification × 40[e], × 400[f]). The patient was treated with chemotherapy to which he appeared to have responded but subsequently developed ascites and recurrent disease and died 1.5 years later. *CT* computed tomography. (C&D: Courtesy of Dr. Florencia G. Que, Mayo Clinic Rochester, MN)

jugular vein thrombosis associated with weight loss, weakness, and anemia; who on workup was found to have peritoneal mesothelioma [38].

Some patients develop a paraneoplastic syndrome after mesothelioma diagnosis. Tanriverdi et al. reported a 51-year-old woman who was diagnosed with malignant pleural mesothelioma and underwent chemotherapy [42]. Two weeks after completion of the chemotherapy, the patient developed anti-Yo-related paraneoplastic cerebellar degeneration. Bech and Sorensen described a 57-year-old man with malignant pleural mesothelioma who developed sensory–motor polyneuropathy 18 days after diagnosis of the mesothelioma [40]. Extensive workup could not identify a specific cause for those symptoms and therefore a paraneoplastic syndrome was suspected. The patient was treated with immunoglobulin and prednisolone with improvement of the symptoms.

Constitutional Symptoms

Malignant mesothelioma patients might present with constitutional symptoms such as fatigue, hyperhidrosis, weight loss, tiredness, or sweating. They may also exhibit dry cough, fever, or night sweats [2]. These symptoms are usually found at advanced stage of the disease. In a study of malignant peritoneal mesotheliomas, vomiting was associated with worse survival [36].

Demographics of Malignant Mesothelioma

Because malignant mesothelioma most commonly is associated with occupational asbestos exposure, the disease is more common in men than in women and more frequent in advanced ages [2]. Therefore, diffuse malignant mesothelioma is usually a disease of adult men.

Overall, malignant pleural mesotheliomas are more common than malignant peritoneal mesotheliomas. Epidemiological studies have shown that peritoneal tumors once comprised approximately 30% of all malignant mesotheliomas [42]; in some case studies, peritoneal mesotheliomas outnumbered pleural mesothelioma. For instance, Ribak et al. [30] studied 2271 consecutive deaths among 17,800 asbestos insulation workers in the USA and Canada (1967–1984); 134 patients had pleural and 222 had peritoneal mesotheliomas. Furthermore, of 86 Swedish insulation workers who died between 1970 and 1994, seven died of malignant peritoneal mesothelioma but none of pleural mesothelioma [43]. However, the percentage of peritoneal mesotheliomas dropped to approximately 7–17% of all mesotheliomas in more recent years [42, 44–46]. This probably is not due to a decreasing incidence of peritoneal mesotheliomas, but rather an increased occurrence of pleural mesothelioma possibly due to an increased intensity of exposure [42].

Because of the relative rarity of pleural mesotheliomas in women, the ratio of peritoneal to pleural mesotheliomas is higher in women (1:2) than in men (1:5) [34].

Malignant Pleural Mesothelioma

Men comprise 60–84% of all cases of malignant pleural mesothelioma [6, 7, 23, 24]. The mean age for men with malignant pleural mesothelioma has been reported between 54 and 59 years with an age range from 20 to 77 years [7, 23]. The mean age for women is very similar and described between 55 and 60 years, ranging from 24 to 80 years [7, 23]. In studies that did not report age by gender, the mean age for malignant pleural mesothelioma was between 51 and 68 years with reported age ranges from 19 to 88 years [6, 24, 30]. However, although rare, malignant pleural mesotheliomas have also been described in children [47, 48].

Malignant Peritoneal Mesothelioma

Similar to diffuse malignant pleural mesotheliomas, peritoneal mesotheliomas are more commonly reported in men than women. In a study of 81 patients with malignant peritoneal mesotheliomas, 57 men (70.4%) and 24 women were included [35]. Acherman et al. [29] reported that out of 51 patients with malignant peritoneal mesothelioma, 34 were men (66.7%).

In a study of 75 malignant peritoneal mesotheliomas in women, the mean age was 47.4 years with an age range from 17 to 92 years [34]. In other studies, the mean age for men was between 51.2 and 63.0 years and for women between 48.7 and 68.0 years [29, 35].

Malignant peritoneal mesotheliomas have rarely been described in children [48, 49].

Laboratory Findings

Pleural Effusion

Effusions in malignant mesothelioma are of exudative quality as established by Light criteria [50] that include one or more of the following: (1) pleural fluid/serum (PF/S) protein ratio greater than 0.5; (2) PF/S lactate dehydrogenase (LDH) greater than 0.6; and (3) pleural fluid LDH level greater than two-thirds of the serum upper limit of normal [51]. Gottherer et al. characterized the pleural fluids of 26 patients with diffuse malignant pleural mesothelioma [52]. (Table 3.3). All pleural fluids

Table 3.3 Characteristics of pleural fluid in malignant pleural mesothelioma based on findings by Gottehrer et al. [52]

Pleural fluid analyte	Mean (range)
Glucose (mg/dL)	75 (13–222)
Glucose PF/S	0.64 (0.1–1.07)
LDH (IU/L)	516 (53–2,364)
LDH PF/S	3.21 (0.55–21.3)
Protein (g/dL)	4.3 (1.9–5.7)
Protein PF/S	0.64 (0.27–0.85)
WBC (per microL)	1,617 (55–10,800)
RBC (per microL)	56,363 (19–560,000)

PF/S pleural fluid/serum ratio, *WBC* white blood cell count, *RBC* red blood cell count

were determined to be exudative by protein and LDH levels. The pleural fluid of nine (of 17) patients had a low pH (<7.30, range 6.92–7.26); in eight patients, the pleural fluid had a pH of ≥7.30. The study showed that patients with lower pleural fluid pH and PF/S glucose ratio had a shorter survival. In a study by Tanrikulu et al., a pleural fluid glucose level of ≤40 mg/dL and a serum LDH level of ≤500 U/L was associated with poor survival [24].

Biomarkers for Malignant Mesothelioma

Research has focused on the identification of serological and fluid markers for diagnosis, response to treatment, and prognosis of malignant mesothelioma. Although some promising candidate markers have been studied, currently, there are no serologic or fluid markers to aid in establishing a diagnosis of malignant mesothelioma because low sensitivity and specificity do not allow for their use in routine clinical practice. However, evidence suggests that some markers might be useful in the follow up of patients after treatment to identify possible recurrence and/or progression of disease. Other markers might have some prognostic value. Some of the more recently studied biomarkers include fibulin-3, mesothelin, and osteopontin.

Fibulin-3 is an extracellular glycoprotein that is encoded by the *epidermal growth factor-containing fibulin-like extracellular matrix protein (EFEMP1)* gene. Recently, Pass et al. showed that plasma and effusion fibulin-3 levels were significantly higher in patients with pleural mesothelioma than in asbestos-exposed people without mesothelioma [53]. These studies concluded that in conjunction with effusion fibulin-3 levels, plasma fibulin-3 levels might be able to differentiate mesothelioma effusions from other malignant and benign effusions. However, additional studies will be required to determine the role of fibulin-3 as a biomarker for diagnosis and monitoring patients after initial treatment.

Mesothelin, a glycoprotein that is expressed on the surface of benign mesothelial cells, was found to be overexpressed in some malignant mesothelioma. Soluble mesothelin-related peptides (SMRPs) are thought to be a splice-variant of mesothelin that can be found in serum and pleural fluid [54]. Elevated levels of SMRP have been identified in epithelioid but not sarcomatoid mesotheliomas. However, mesothelin can also be increased in other tumors such as ovarian carcinoma, pancreatic carcinoma, and lung cancers or in renal insufficiency. Furthermore, the sensitivity and specificity appear to depend on the detection method and cutoff values used and therefore, further studies are necessary to establish the diagnostic and prognostic importance of that biomarker.

Osteopontin is a glycoprotein that mediates cell–matrix interactions and is overexpressed in several types of cancers. Pass et al. showed that serum osteopontin levels were significantly higher in patients with malignant pleural mesothelioma than in patients with exposure to asbestos [55]. Furthermore, tumor cells stained for osteopontin in 36 of 38 cases of pleural mesothelioma. However, further studies are necessary to confirm those data.

Carcinoembryonic antigen (CEA) has also been studied for its use in malignant mesothelioma. A meta-analysis of 11 studies that identified the value of CEA to distinguish between malignant mesothelioma and metastatic lung cancer showed that the sensitivity of CEA for malignant pleural mesothelioma ranged from 0.73 to 1.00 (mean 0.97, 95% CI: 0.93–0.99) when the CEA assay was negative [56]. Interestingly, in 8 of 11 studies the sensitivities were 1.00 and only one study showed a relative low sensitivity (0.73). Therefore, a high pleural fluid CEA might assist in ruling out malignant mesothelioma, and the pleural fluid CEA assay might be useful in helping distinguish malignant pleural mesothelioma from metastatic lung cancer.

Hyaluronic acid (HA) has been proposed as a putative diagnostic marker because its level is increased in approximately 60% of pleural effusions from patients with malignant mesothelioma [57]. On the other hand, Fuhrman et al. did not show a significant difference in HA of pleural fluid between benign pleural effusion and effusion associated with malignant pleural mesothelioma; however, HA was significantly higher in mesothelioma than in nonmesothelioma malignancies [58]. In the serum, elevated HA levels have been described only in advanced stage mesothelioma [59]; and a significant percentage of malignant mesothelioma may not secrete HA [58, 60].

Studies suggest that a combination of biomarkers might be superior to the use of any single marker. Creaney et al. showed that a combination of effusion HA, and serum and effusion mesothelin had a greater diagnostic accuracy than effusion mesothelin alone [61]. Furthermore, SMRP might improve CYFRA-21–1 and CEA accuracy in pleural effusion in the differential diagnosis of malignant pleural mesothelioma [62]. Further studies are necessary to identify a combination of biomarkers that might be helpful in the diagnosis, prognosis, and disease progression of malignant mesothelioma.

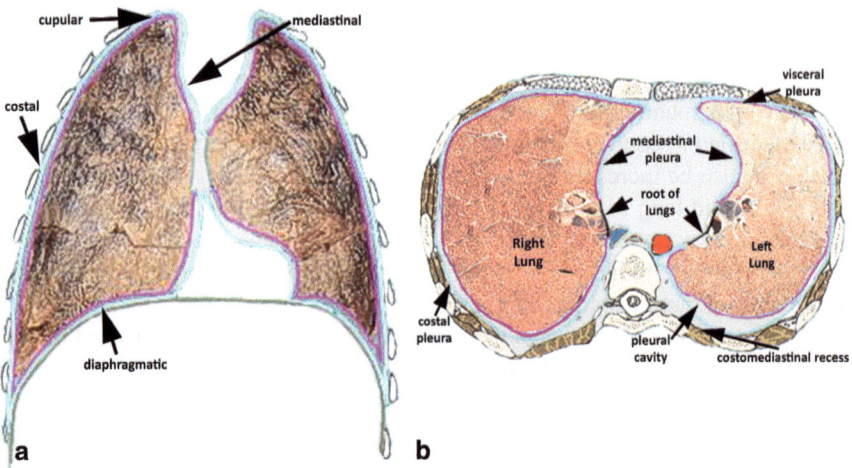

Fig. 3.3 Schematic images illustrate the gross anatomic locations of pleural anatomy (**a**) and the relationships of the parietal (*blue*) and visceral *(purple)* pleura to each other. The anteroposterior relationship of this anatomy is shown in (**b**) and correlates with what is seen on conventional axial CT image acquisitions. *CT* computed tomography. (Reprinted with permission of Dr. Wesley Norman, "The Anatomy Lesson," 1999)

Clinical and Radiological Staging of Malignant Pleural Mesothelioma

Staging of malignant pleural mesothelioma sets the stage for therapeutic management and overall outcome. Radiologic staging, as such, involves a pattern search that is based largely on pleural anatomy which is not necessarily straightforward. Pleural anatomy is grossly partitioned into the cupola or cervical pleura, the mediastinal pleura, the costal pleura, and the diaphragmatic pleura [63, 64]. The cervical pleura surrounds the apices of the lungs and can extend into the neck as much as 5 cm above the sternal end of the first rib. The mediastinal pleura adheres to the pericardium with phrenic nerve coursing between them. The costal pleura lies immediately adjacent to loose connective tissue called the endothoracic fascia which abuts the thoracic wall (the sternum, costal cartilages, ribs, and chest wall muscles), and the diaphragmatic pleura covers the diaphragm except for the central tendon. The inferior aspect of the pleura extends to the T12 vertebral body with the approximate inferior extent of the pleura being about two fingerbreadths inferior to the lung. Posteriorly, the pleura is reflected upon the side of the vertebral bodies. (Fig. 3.3a, b)

Knowledge of pleural lymphatic drainage is helpful in radiological staging. Lymphatic drainage of the visceral pleura and the lung are the same; however, lymphatic drainage of the parietal pleura can be complex. The anterior parietal pleura drains into the internal mammary lymph nodes. The posterior parietal pleura drains into paraspinal lymph nodes. Anteriorly, the diaphragmatic pleura drains into internal mammary and anterior diaphragmatic lymph nodes while posteriorly, it drains into para-aortic and posterior mediastinal lymph nodes. In the setting of suspected malignant pleural mesothelioma, any lymph nodes in the extrapleural space are best viewed with suspicion.

The present TNM (tumor, node, metastasis) system (Table 3.4) is based on the largest, multicenter and international database on malignant pleural mesothelioma from the International Association for the Study of Lung Cancer (IASLC), and is able to classify patients into different outcomes [65–67]. Using the TNM descriptors, staging of malignant pleural mesothelioma has been established (Table 3.5) [65].

Analysis of the IASLC database has shown that the survival of malignant pleural mesothelioma is significantly affected by the overall tumor stage ($p<0.0001$), T classification ($p<0.0001$), N classification ($p<0.0001$), tumor histology ($p<0.0001$), patient gender ($p=0.0002$) and age ($p=0.0025$), and type of operation (curative versus palliative, $p<0.0001$) [66]. Also shown in that analysis were statistically significant differences in survival between adjacent paired stages (except stage I vs. II), adjacent paired T categories (except T1 vs. T2), and adjacent paired N categories (except N1 vs. N2). Currently, clinical outcome depends a great deal on the ability of imaging to distinguish between stages II and III, III and IV, or between T2 and T3, or T3 and T4 disease, or between N0 and N1, or N2 and N3 disease. Distinction between potentially resectable (T3) and unresectable (T4) disease remains challenging, and unfortunately, as detailed below, limitations of imaging have not precluded the need for surgical staging to make this decision.

Radiologic Features

The primary role of imaging in malignant mesotheliomas lies in preoperative staging and assessment of treatment response, disease recurrence, or metastasis. Initial screening of the chest, regardless of clinical suspicion, often begins with a chest radiograph, largely due to accessibility and lower cost. Chest radiographs, depending on the number of views, generally cost around US$ 150–200. Additional characterization with cross-sectional imaging techniques, more often with CT than with magnetic resonance imaging (MRI) or positron emission tomography/computer tomography (PET/CT) are also performed with varying degrees of sensitivity and specificity. At present, a CT costs roughly US$ 1500; and, MRI and PET/CT are more expensive with an MRI costing about twice that of a CT and a PET/CT about twice that of an MRI. Of the cross-sectional imaging modalities, CT is most frequently obtained, again largely because of accessibility and cost when compared to PET/CT and MRI. Ultrasonography, another cross-sectional imaging technique, has been used but it is generally performed for targeted evaluation given the superior coverage afforded by the other imaging modalities. Endobronchial ultrasound or EBUS is performed by interventional pulmonologists and is not included in this section.

Table 3.4 The international association for the study of lung cancer (IASLC) malignant pleural mesothelioma staging system

T—Primary tumor	
T1	
T1a	Tumor limited to ipsilateral parietal pleura, including mediastinal and diaphragmatic pleura; no involvement of the visceral pleura
T1b	Tumor involving the ipsilateral parietal pleura including mediastinal and diaphragmatic pleura; scattered foci of tumor also involving visceral pleura
T2	
	Tumor involving each of the ipsilateral pleural surfaces (visceral, parietal, mediastinal, and diaphragmatic) with at least one of the following features:
	Involvement of diaphragmatic muscle
	Confluent visceral pleural tumor (including fissures), or extension of tumor from visceral pleura into underlying pulmonary parenchyma
T3 Locally advanced but potentially resectable tumor	
	Tumor involving all of the ipsilateral pleural surfaces (visceral, parietal, mediastinal and diaphragmatic) with at least one of the following features:
	Involvement of endothoracic fascia
	Extension into mediastinal fat
	Solitary, completely resectable focus of tumor extending into the soft tissues of the chest wall
	Non-transmural involvement of the pericardium
T4 Locally advanced technically unresectable tumor	
	Tumor involving all of the ipsilateral pleural surfaces (visceral, parietal, mediastinal and diaphragmatic) with at least one of the following:

3 Clinical and Radiologic Features

Table 3.4 (continued)

T—Primary tumor	
	Diffuse extension or multifocal masses of tumor in the chest wall, with or without associated rib destruction
	Direct transdiaphragmatic extension of tumor to the peritoneum
	Direct extension of tumor to the contralateral pleura
	Direct extension of tumor to one or more mediastinal organs
	Direct extension of tumor into the spine
	Tumor extending through the pericardium to internal surface of pericardium with or without pericardial effusion; or tumor involving the myocardium
N—Lymph nodes	
NX	Regional lymph nodes cannot be assessed
N0	No regional lymph node metastases
N1	Metastases in ipsilateral bronchopulmonary or hilar lymph nodes
N2	Metastases in subcarinal or ipsilateral mediastinal lymph nodes, including ipsilateral internal mammary nodes
N3	Metastases in contralateral mediastinal, contralateral internal mammary, ipsilateral or contralateral supraclavicular lymph nodes
M—Metastases	
MX	Distant metastases cannot be assessed
M0	No distant metastases
M1	Distant metastases present

Table 3.5 Clinical and TNM staging of malignant pleural mesothelioma

Stage	Tumor	Node	Metastasis
Ia	T1a	N0	M0
Ib	T1b	N0	M0
II	T2	N0	M0
III	Any T3	Any N1 or N2	M0
IV	Any T4	Any N3	Any M1

Chest Radiographs

Conventional chest radiograph provides two views of the chest, a posterior–anterior (PA) view and a lateral view. In the absence of pleural disease, the pleura is generally appreciated simply as the "edge" of the relatively radiolucent lungs. Pleural disease usually manifests as circumferential pleural thickening that often has better conspicuity where the X-ray beams are perpendicular to the pleura—laterally and medially on the PA view and anteriorly and posterior on the lateral view. Radiographic appearances of pleural disease are quite variable and can include a normal appearance particularly in early disease, pleural thickening (focal, diffuse, or nodular), pleural effusion, pleural mass, or complete hemithorax opacification (Fig. 3.4). When the pleura is diffusely thickened, a rind of soft tissue often has a nodular or scalloped appearance that becomes more obvious with more advanced disease (Fig. 3.5). A single anterior–posterior (AP) chest radiograph is generally performed on hospitalized patients who are unable to

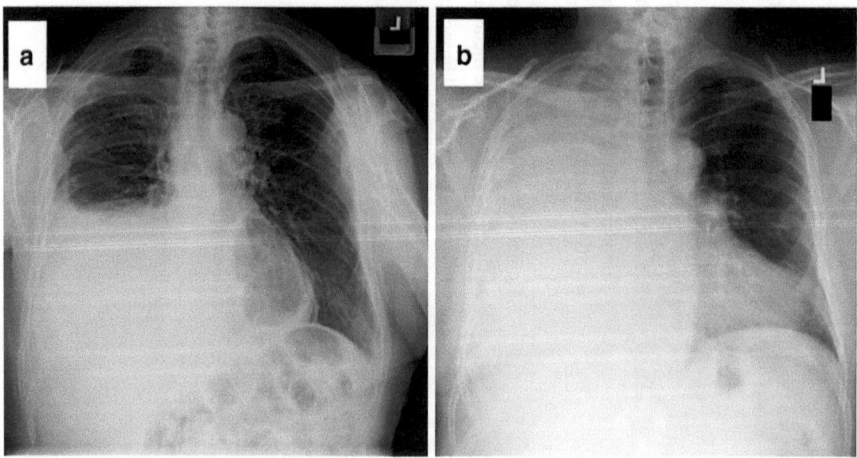

Fig. 3.4 Two different patients with malignant pleural mesothelioma illustrating unilateral right-sided pleural effusion. In **a**, there is a moderate to large pleural effusion and pleural thickening. In **b**, opacification of the right hemithorax is not associated with significant mediastinal shift; in particular, there is no significant mediastinal shift toward the opacification. Differential considerations include mass (pleural, chest wall, or pulmonary), pleural effusion, and consolidation

3 Clinical and Radiologic Features

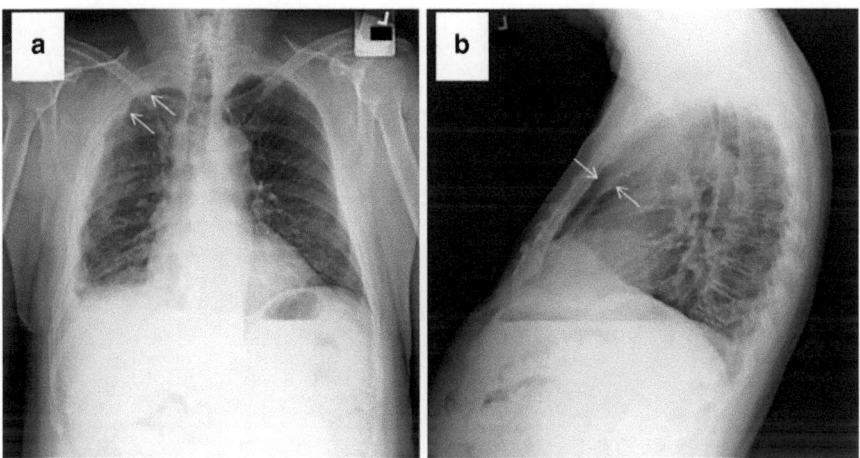

Fig. 3.5 Posterior–anterior (**a**) and lateral (**b**) chest radiographs of the same patient with malignant pleural mesothelioma. Note the nodular pleural thickening that partially encases the right lung (*arrows*) which has relative decreased lung volume compared to the left lung. On the lateral view (**b**), the nodular pleural thickening is best appreciated anteriorly (*arrows*). Notice also the lucent left costophrenic angle but blunted right costophrenic angle which could be from pleural thickening or fluid

assume an upright position (Fig. 3.6). How much the patient is "propped up" is generally indicated on the film. The radiographic signs that suggest early disease include asymmetric volume loss of the involved lung over the contralateral one (in the setting of unilateral disease; Fig. 3.7), and unilateral pleural effusion.

Computed Tomography

CT is the primary workhorse in imaging evaluation of malignant mesothelioma. Many of the CT features described for malignant mesothelioma over a decade ago [68] still apply today. There remains great variability in the pleural CT imaging features of malignant pleural mesothelioma, ranging from nonspecific plaques (noncalcified and calcified) to focal masses to diffuse irregular or nodular pleural thickening encasing the entire lung. (Fig. 3.8) With CT, more detailed assessment of the chest wall, pericardium, mediastinum, diaphragm, and major vessels can be made. In a study of 215 patients with pleural disease, 99 of which with malignant pleural mesothelioma, multivariate analysis resulted in three CT findings for differentiating mesothelioma from metastatic pleural disease; these included (i) rind-like pleural involvement (sensitivity/specificity 70/85 %), (ii) mediastinal pleural involvement (sensitivity/specificity 85/67 %), and (iii) pleural thickness more than 1 cm (sensitivity/specificity 59/82 %) [69]. Evidence of unilateral volume loss can be supported by elevation of the ipsilateral hemidiaphragm, ipsilateral shift of the mediastinum, and narrowing of the intercostal spaces.

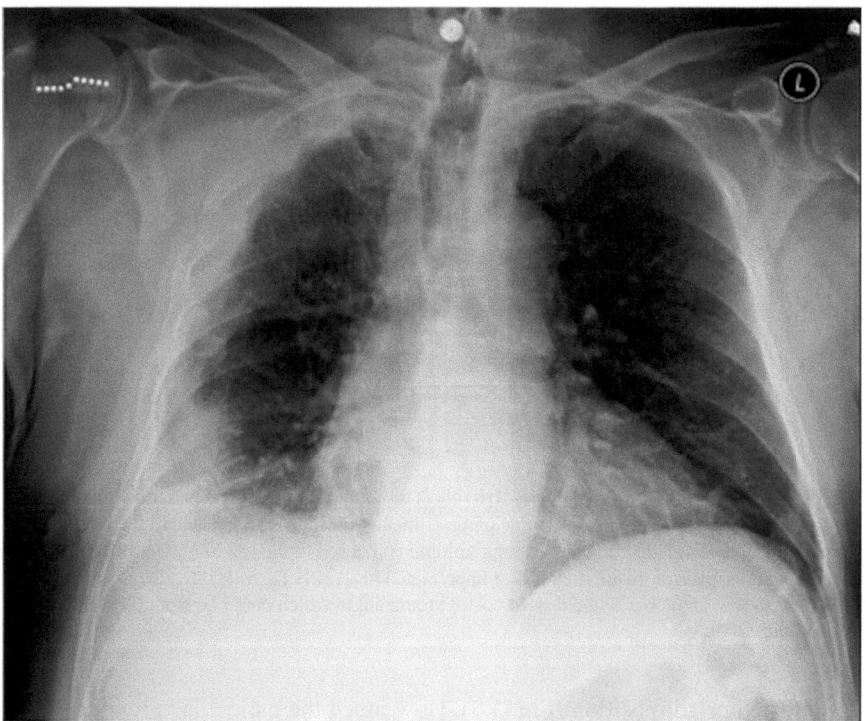

Fig. 3.6 Anterior–posterior chest radiograph of the same patient as in Fig. 3.4, who was later hospitalized. Note the indicator for the degree of inclination projected over the upper right humeral head. Notice nodular pleural thickening on the right and the relatively smaller right lung compared to the left

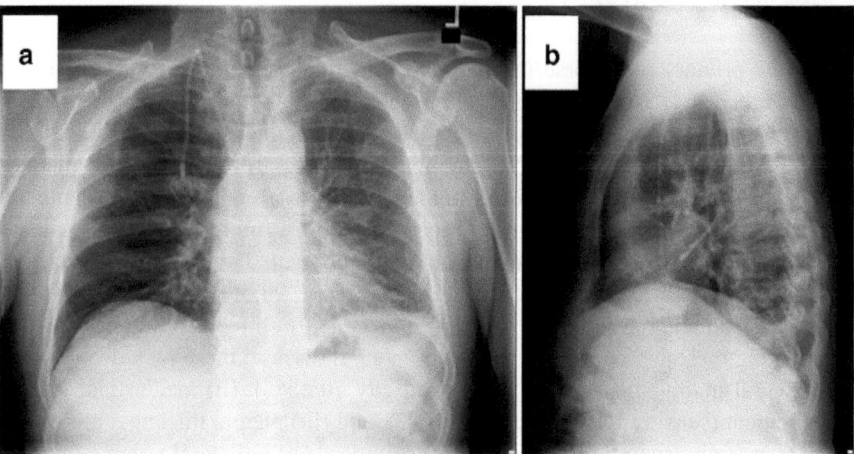

Fig. 3.7 Chest radiograph—posterior–anterior (**a**) and lateral (**b**)—shows a small left pleural effusion and decreased left lung volume compared to the right. There is also left pleural thickening

3 Clinical and Radiologic Features

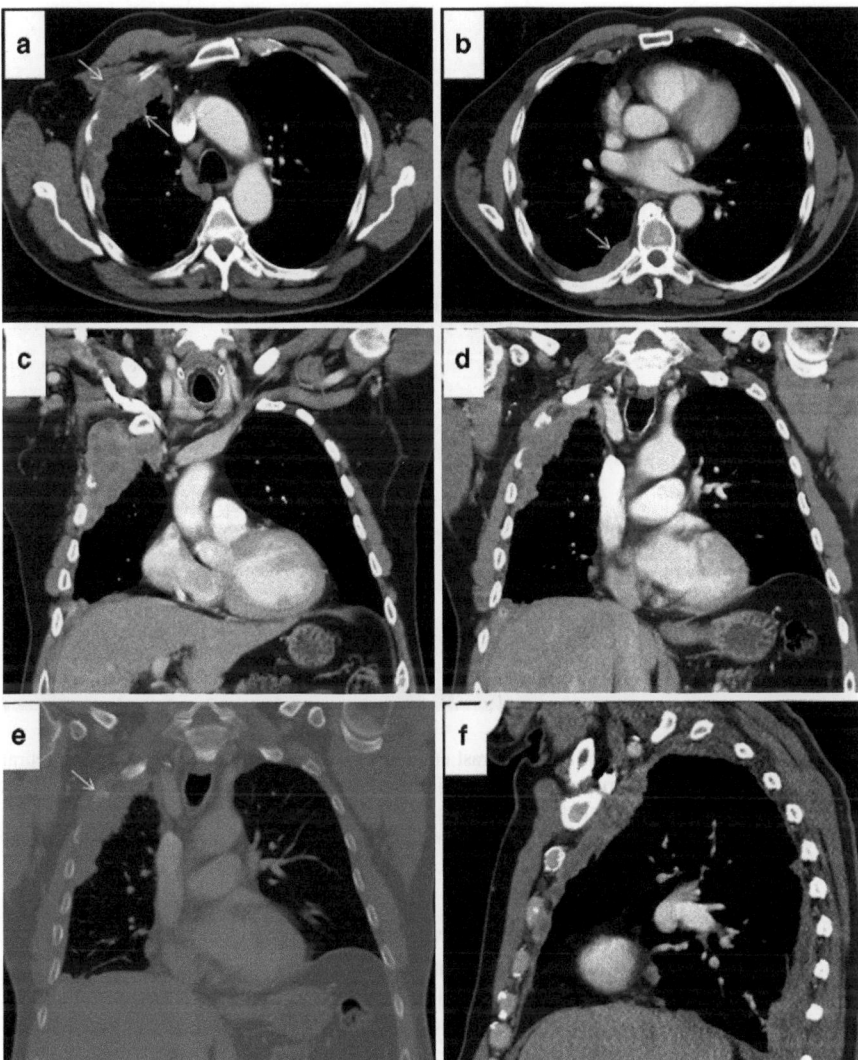

Fig. 3.8 Contrast-enhanced chest CT axial images (**a, b**) of a patient with malignant pleural mesothelioma demonstrate nodular pleural thickening on the right (*arrows*). Coronal reformatted views (**c, d**) show extension of the anterolateral component of the pleural thickening into the chest wall with destruction of the overlying ribs which are confirmed on bone windows (*arrow*) (**e**). A sagittal reformatted view (**f**) offers another opportunity to assess for the extent of disease. *CT* computed tomography

CT can be performed with or without intravenous iodinated contrast. Often, intravenous contrast is administered in the setting of malignant mesothelioma because the additional soft tissue contrast and enhanced conspicuity of details generally can help the radiologist assess for effacement of fatty planes by infiltrative disease at the mediastinal (particularly pericardial), diaphragmatic, pleural, and chest wall levels.

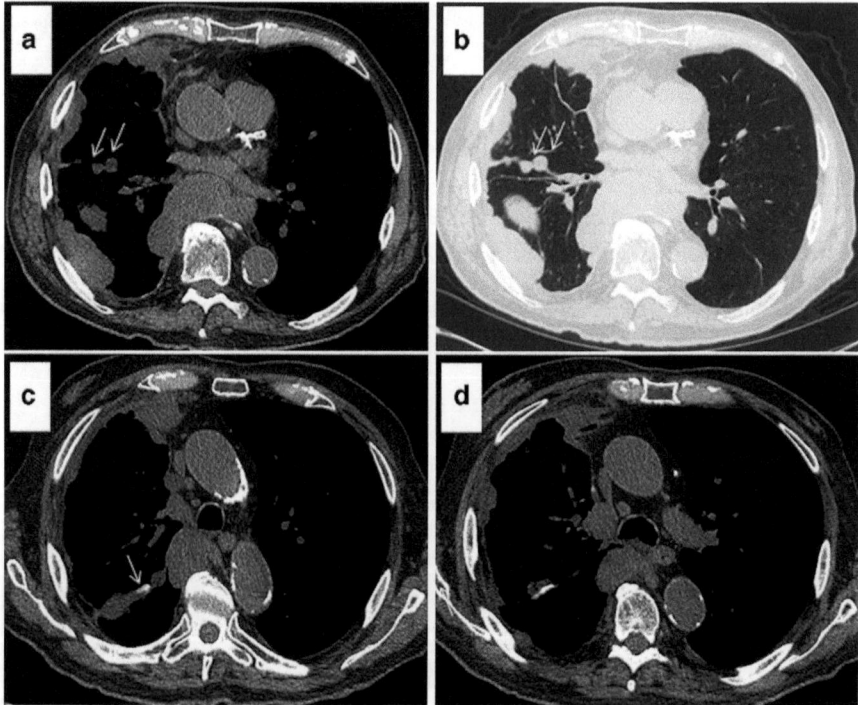

Fig. 3.9 A single axial slice of a noncontrast enhanced CT **a** of a patient with malignant pleural mesothelioma, including corresponding lung windows **b** demonstrates nodular pleural thickening on the right side that extends into the right major fissure (*arrows*). The right lung volume is smaller than the left. Two other axial slices **c, d** show nodular pleural thickening with associated calcifications (*arrow*), also extending into the right major fissure. *CT* computed tomography

Another use of intravenous contrast, particularly as a way to assess hemodynamic function or perfusion of disease, is still at an investigatory stage [70].

Determination of parietal involvement by disease is important in staging. Despite the very high in-plane resolution of CT, the distinction between normal visceral and parietal pleura is extremely challenging; the distinction is much easier in the setting of pleural effusion and sometimes in the setting of pleural masses. An investigation into using Hounsfield units, which indicate CT attenuation or radiodensity of the image pixels, has shown that malignant pleural mesothelioma soft tissue tends to have Hounsfield units that fall between pleural effusion and muscle and liver [71]. This overlap makes it challenging for imaging to adequately distinguish the extent of disease, particularly across tissue planes. Without intravenous contrast and even in some cases with intravenous contrast, the soft tissue contrast differences between pleura, endothoracic fascia, and even chest wall can be nearly impossible to ascertain with certainty. Involvement of the interlobar fissural pleura is characteristic of mesothelioma (Fig. 3.9) and can be sometimes more apparent on reformatted sagittal or coronal views compared to the conventional axial views.

CT staging of malignant pleural mesothelioma for extrapleural involvement includes the chest wall with particular attention to the ribs and spine, the mediastinum with particular attention to the pericardium and extension into the contralateral hemithorax, lymph node involvement including the hilar, middle mediastinal, internal mammary, anterior diaphragmatic regions, as well as hemidiaphragmatic involvement with particular attention to transdiaphragmatic involvement. The literature has shown high sensitivity (>90%) of both CT and MRI in the ability to assess for resectability especially for evaluation of the chest wall, mediastinum, and diaphragm [72] but the specificity of these imaging studies is more disappointing. Detection of diaphragmatic invasion is still challenging by CT, and while MRI can provide additional information, surgical staging in this region is often warranted.

Magnetic Resonance Imaging

MRI uses a nonionizing technique for image acquisition, and patients loosely know it as the "no radiation" scan. MRI provides exquisite soft tissue detail and contrast, and the physical phenomenon measured with the MRI technique can give some insight into the nature of the soft tissue make-up of its components. Multiplanar acquisitions widen imaging approaches and cardiac gated and respiratory compensation techniques reduce much of the motion artifacts which used to preclude diagnostic use of MRI in the chest. In a prospective study, CT and MRI were nearly equivalent in diagnostic accuracy of staging; however, MRI was superior to CT in revealing diaphragmatic invasion, endothoracic fascia invasion, and in showing solitary resectable foci of chest wall invasion [73]. The different T1 and T2 relaxivities of soft tissues are accentuated on T1-weighted and T2-weighted non-contrast-enhanced techniques. Malignant pleural mesothelioma tends to have slightly higher T2 signal which is accentuated with fat suppression (Fig. 3.10). With intravenous gadolinium-based contrast agents, some of the soft tissue detail is accentuated (Fig. 3.11).

Diffusion-weighted imaging (DWI) is an MRI technique that reflects the degree of Brownian motion of the protons (essentially from water molecules) within soft tissue. As such, water protons whose diffusivity is restricted by increased cellularity (such as in malignancies) or by debris or macromolecules (such as in abscesses) will be higher signaling on diffusion-weighted imaging (Fig. 3.12). The restricted diffusivity of these protons is reflected in a quantitative metric called the apparent diffusion coefficient (ADC). Initial experience with DWI at 3T has shown promise for differentiating malignant pleural disease from benign disease with improvement of sensitivity with dynamic contrast-enhanced MRI [74]. The "pointillism sign" described as hypersignaling foci on DWI obtained at high diffusion sensitivities or b-values (Fig. 3.13) is thought to be caused by multifocal deposits of tumor [74]. This suggests that this might be a way for targeted biopsy, but ongoing investigation continues in this area.

Imaging assessment for disease progression or treatment response is challenging in malignant pleural mesothelioma. A modified response evaluation criteria in solid tumor (RECIST) approach for measuring such disease [75] is available given interobserver and intraobserver variability and is often used in clinical trials and staging protocols as well as in evaluating treatment response. Investigations continue on volume measurements of disease from imaging [76]. Fast image acquisi-

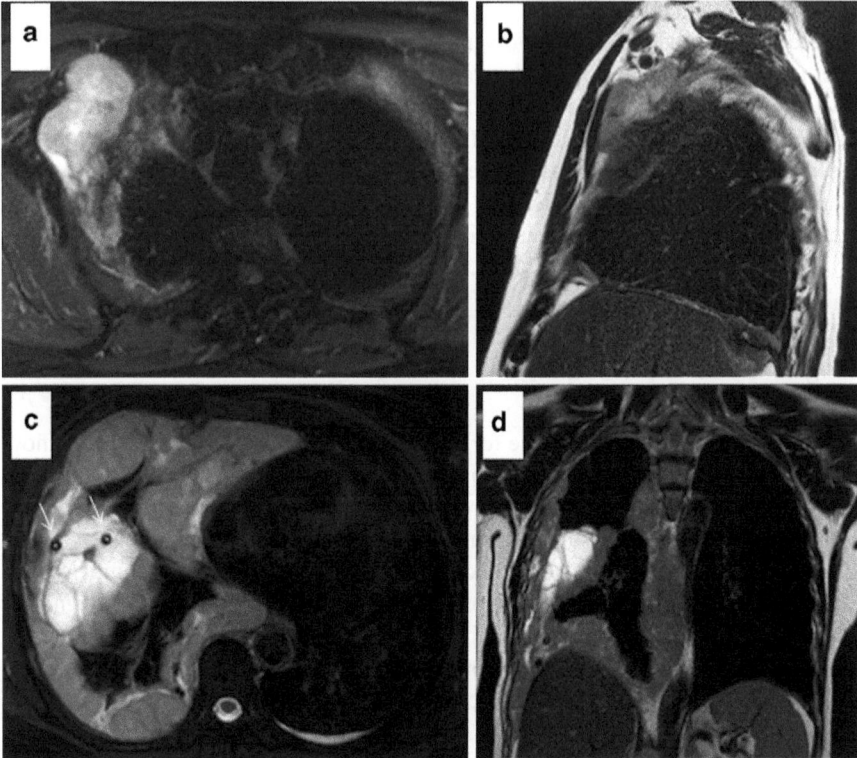

Fig. 3.10 Multiplanar T2-weighted MRI acquisitions of two patients with malignant pleural mesothelioma. Axial fat-suppressed T2-weighted image **a** of one patient demonstrates pleural nodularity on the right side that extends into the chest wall where it appears as a lobulated mass with some central necrosis. Sagittal nonfat suppressed T2-weighted image acquisition **b** of the same patient shows soft tissue signaling distinction between the chest wall mass, the overlying muscles, and the adjacent fat. In a different patient with malignant pleural mesothelioma, axial fat-suppressed T2-weighted image **c** demonstrates a thickened nodular pleural "rind" on the right side, loculated, complex, septated pleural fluid, and two round susceptibility artifacts (*arrows*) consistent with parts of a chest tube. A coronal non-fat-suppressed T2 weighted image (**d**) shows soft tissue contrasts between the thickened pleura and the hemidiaphragm. *MRI* magnetic resonance imaging

tion techniques, such as steady state free precession sequences, are fast enough to acquire images while the patient is breathing. Images acquired in this manner allow for evaluation of hemidiaphragmatic motion which can be limited by diaphragmatic tumor invasion or by disease invading the phrenic nerve.

Positron Emission Tomography/Computer Tomography

With its ability to provide information on tumoral metabolic activity as well as anatomic information, PET/CT has been useful in distinguishing benign from malig-

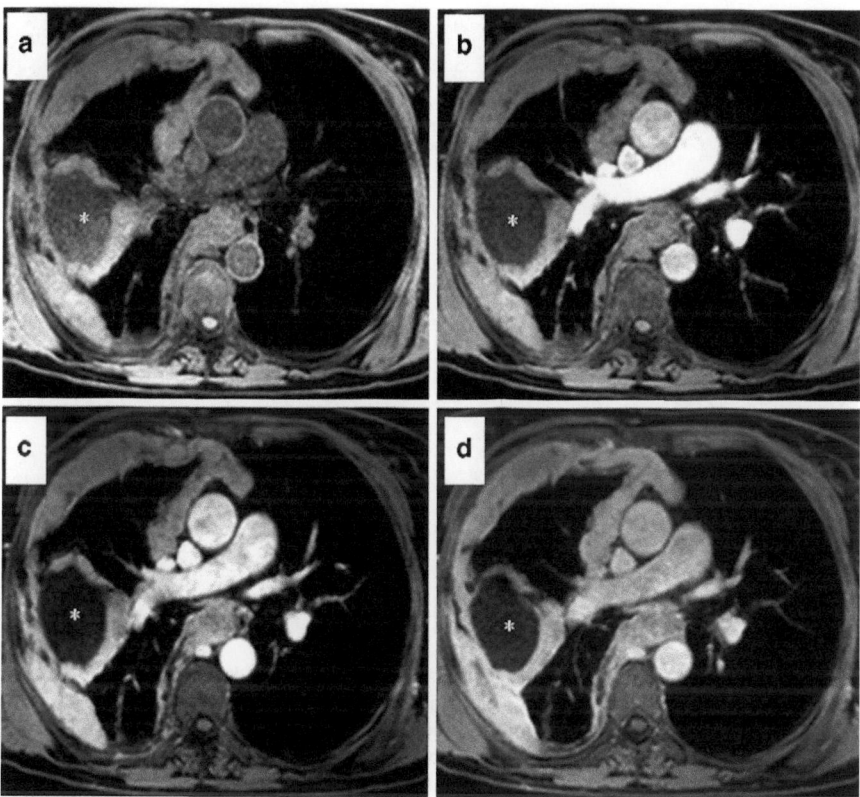

Fig. 3.11 Axial MRI acquisition before intravenous contrast administration (**a**) and three image acquisitions obtained at three different time points after contrast administration (**b–d**; i.e., dynamic contrast-enhanced MRI) demonstrate mostly persistent enhancement of the thickened pleura on the right. The loculated pleural effusion (*) which was seen on Fig. 3.9c shows no enhancement. *MRI* magnetic resonance imaging

nant pleural disease and in the staging, post-therapeutic follow-up, and prognosis of malignant pleural mesothelioma [70, 77–79] (Fig. 3.14). In 63 consecutive patients with histologically proven malignant pleural disease, the sensitivity of PET/CT for detecting malignancy was 96.8% with a negative predictive value of 93.9%, while its specificity was 88.5% and its positive predictive value was 93.8% [80]. Various investigations have shown that its primary advantage is one of identifying distant metastases. Standardized uptake values or SUVs are metrics that provide the relative tissue/organ uptake. Despite a relatively large degree of variability of SUVs due to biological, physical, processing, and acquisition errors, SUVs as a form of molecular imaging can facilitate therapy monitoring as well as management decisions [81, 82]. PET/CT plays are large role in the imaging evaluation of malignant pleural mesothelioma, but it, too, is limited in its ability to specify disease infiltrating across tissue planes, often requiring surgical staging or assessment.

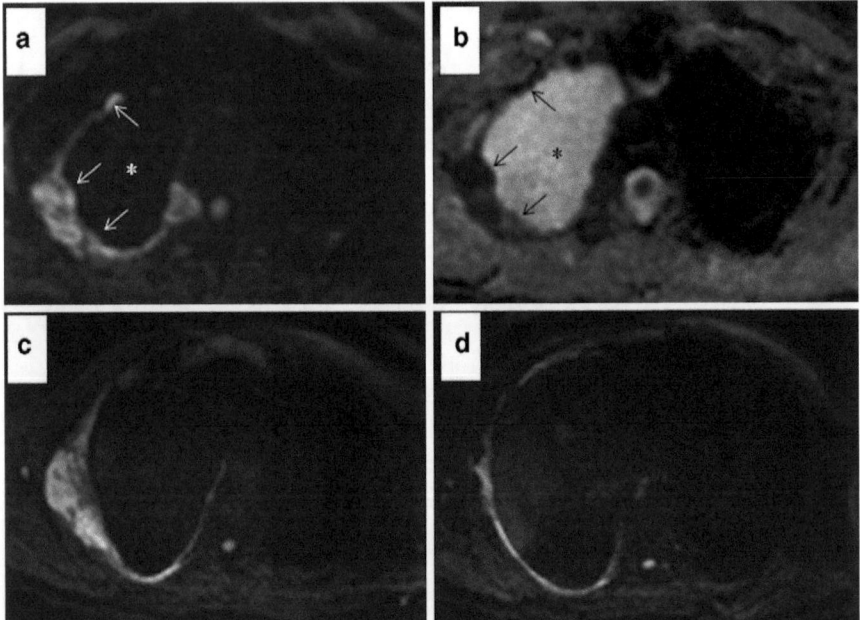

Fig. 3.12 Diffusion-weighted image acquired at b=800 s/mm² (**a**) demonstrates restricted diffusion of the nodular pleural thickening on the right (*arrows*). This finding corresponds to areas of decreased signal on the apparent diffusion coefficient map (**b**). Notice that the signal from the known right pleural effusion (*) has been suppressed on the diffusion-weighted image (**a**) and there is no corresponding low signal on the apparent diffusion coefficient map (**b**). Two additional axial diffusion-weighted images at different locations (**c–d**) demonstrate the rind of restricted diffusion involving the pleura on the right

Ultrasonography

Ultrasonography is a useful technique particularly for targeted evaluation of the pleura. When a pleural effusion is present, it provides an acoustic window which can improve characterization of pleural and even lung findings. Ultrasound-guided thoracenteses as well as percutaneous or transthoracic ultrasound-guided biopsies of pleural masses or thickening are established safe techniques. Ultrasonographic guidance is as effective as CT guidance for transthoracic biopsies with histologic diagnoses achieving greater than 90 % accuracy [83, 84].

Radiological Differential Diagnoses

Many papers have investigated distinguishing between malignant and benign pleural diseases radiologically and although there are a few features that are more suggestive of malignancy, there are a host of other pleural processes besides malig-

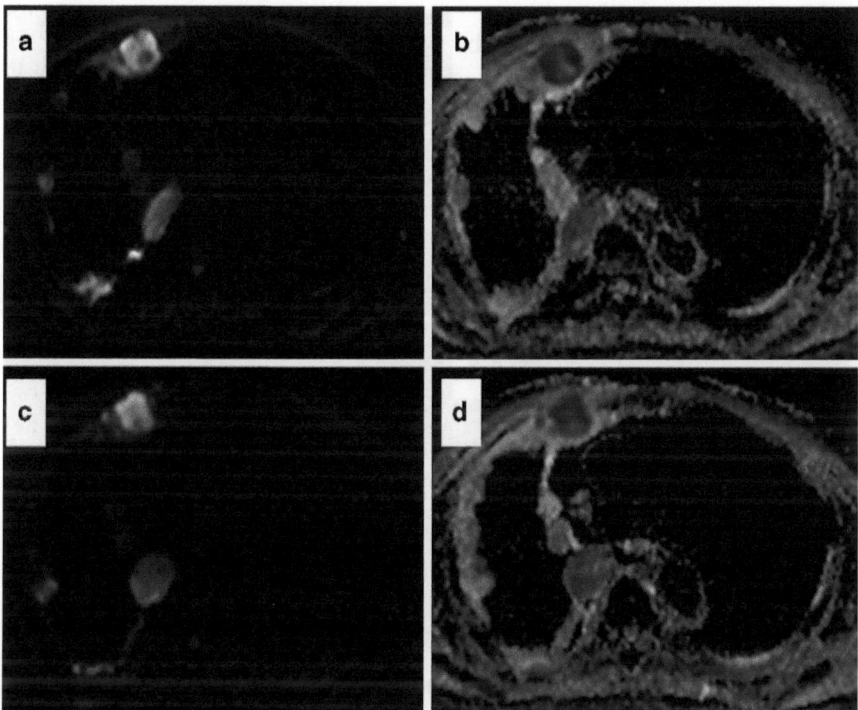

Fig. 3.13 Axial diffusion-weighted imaging and apparent diffusion-coefficient imaging pairs (**a, b** and **c, d**) at two different locations demonstrate nodular right pleural thickening with focal areas of restricted diffusion. These focal areas of restricted diffusion illustrate the pointillism sign and are suggestive of multifocal deposits of disease

nant pleural mesothelioma which should be on the differential diagnoses. These include but are not limited to solid pleural metastases, fibrous tumor of the pleura, asbestos-related diffuse pleural thickening, pleural fibrosis, and invasive thymoma. Other entities that are lower on the differential list include rounded atelectasis, and pleurodesis.

Cases to Illustrate Radiologic and Clinical Features

Case 1

A 74-year-old man presented with recurrent symptomatic right pleural effusion associated with significant right-sided chest pain and dyspnea. He was a never smoker with possible prior exposure to asbestos when he served in the military several decades ago. A CT obtained to assess for coronary artery calcifications showed a small right pleural effusion in addition to coronary artery calcifications (Fig. 3.15a, b). A

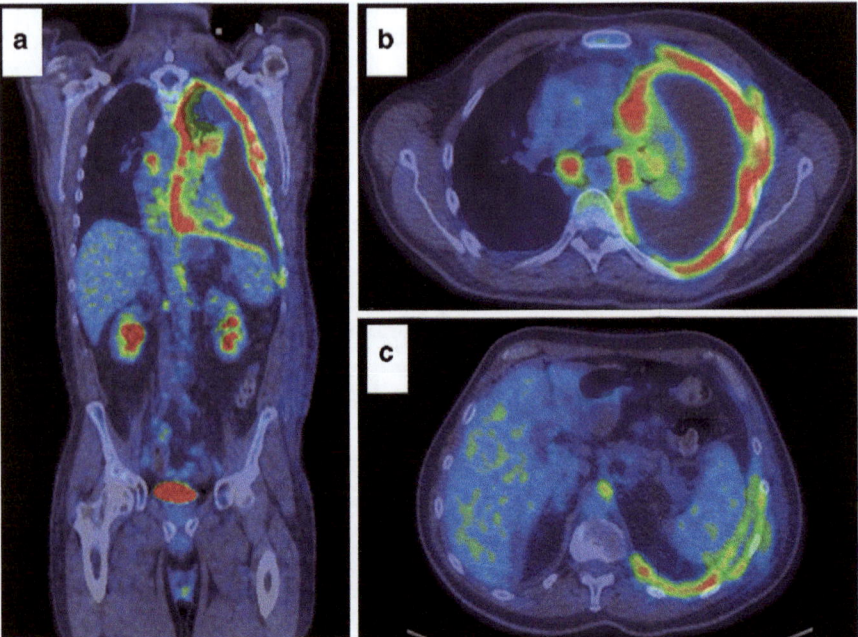

Fig. 3.14 Coronal PET/CT (**a**) and two axial slices (**b, c**) show extensive markedly FDG-avid nodular left pleural thickening encasing the left lung. Also seen on PET are FDG-avid right hilar, right infrahilar, and subcarinal lymph nodes indicating contralateral thoracic spread of disease, as well as FDG-avid upper retroperitoneal and right para-aortic lymph nodes consistent with nodal metastases below the diaphragm. A large left pleural effusion is associated with complete collapse of the left lung and resulting mediastinal shift to the right. *FDG* fluorodeoxyglucose, *PET/CT* positron emission tomography/computer tomography

chest radiograph about a year later demonstrated increase in the right pleural effusion and CT showed increased pleural nodularity (Fig. 3.15c–f). The patient subsequently underwent thoracentesis and cytology demonstrated atypical cells. About 1 month later, PET/CT (Fig. 3.15g, h) was obtained and pleuroscopy was performed (Fig. 3.15i, j) with biopsy. The morphologic and immunophenotypic features were consistent with malignant mesothelioma, epithelioid type (Fig. 3.15k, l). The patient expired 25 days later, about 2.5 years after the initial CT.

Case 2

A 59-year-old man presented with a positive TB skin test during a general medical examination. He has no current symptoms and chest radiograph (Fig. 3.16a, b) was normal. One year later, the patient presented with a new right pleural effusion (Fig. 3.16c, d). Nine months later, right pleural masses are identified on follow-up chest radiographs (Fig. 3.16e, f). A CT was obtained (Fig. 3.16g–j) and the diagnosis

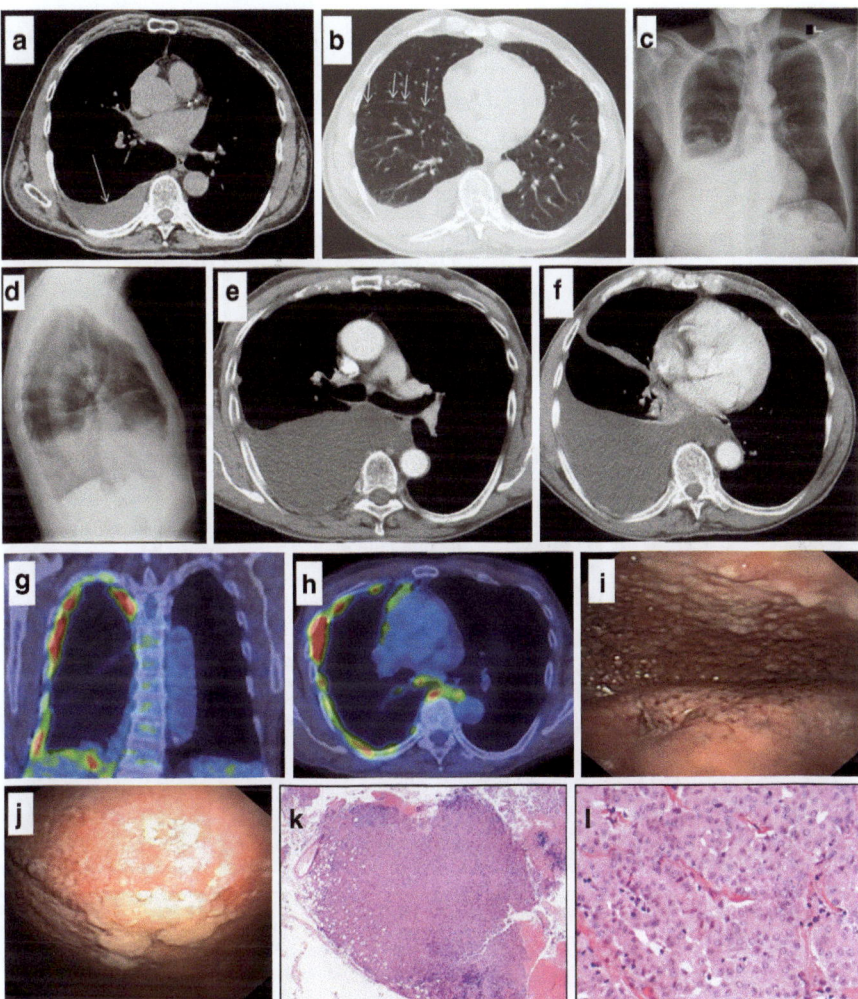

Fig. 3.15 CT without intravenous contrast demonstrates a small right pleural effusion (**a**, *arrow*) and small nodularities (**b**, *arrows*) along the major fissure. Chest radiographs PA (**c**) and lateral (**d**) show an increase in the right pleural effusion and CT (**e**, **f**) demonstrates an increase in the right pleural effusion and increasing pleural nodularity. PET/CT showed extensive nodular hypermetabolic activity involving most of the right pleura (**g**, **h**). Pleuroscopic images (**i**, **j**) demonstrate diffuse nodularity involving the entirety of the parietal pleura. Evaluation also revealed involvement of focal aspects of the visceral pleura, as well as the involvement of the diaphragmatic and mediastinal pleura. Low power view of an H&E slide from a right pleural biopsy reveals sheets of atypical epithelioid cells invading into adipose tissue (**k**). These atypical cells are characterized by ample eosinophilic cytoplasm and round nuclei with prominent nucleoli (**l**). (Magnification x 40 [k], x 400 [l]. The neoplastic cells are positive for calretinin, CK5/6, and WT-1 and lack staining for TTF-1, MOC-31, and BerEp4 (not shown). The morphologic features and immunophenotype are diagnostic of malignant mesothelioma, epithelioid type. *PET/CT* positron emission tomography/computer tomography. (I&J: Courtesy of Dr. John J. Mullon, Mayo Clinic Rochester, MN)

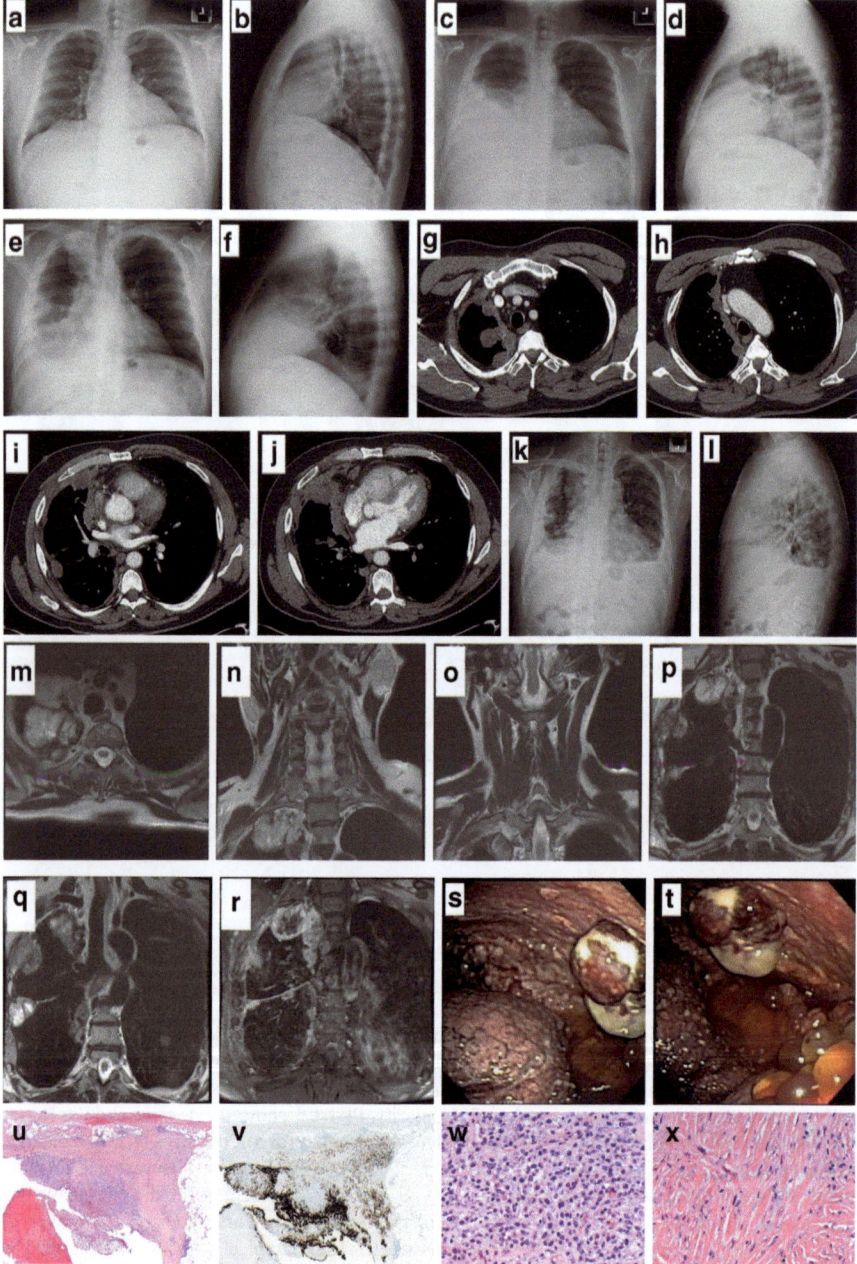

Fig. 3.16 At the time of the positive TB skin test of this 58-year-old man, PA (**a**) and lateral (**b**) chest radiographs were normal. One year later, the patient complained about a cough. Chest radiographs at that time (**c, d**) demonstrated a new moderate to large right pleural effusion with associated atelectasis and consolidation of the right mid and lower lung. Chest radiographs 9 months later demonstrated right pleural masses (**e, f**). Note their development from the prior two chest radiographs. Contrast-enhanced CT (**g–j**) shows circumferential lobulated right pleural thickening

of malignant pleural mesothelioma was established. Chest radiographs (Fig. 3.16k, l) 6 months later showed progression of disease. An MRI of the cervical and thoracic spines (Fig. 3.16m–r) obtained around the same time provided additional characterization of the pleural disease. Pleuroscopy was performed (Fig. 3.16s, t). A biopsy of the parietal pleura revealed biphasic malignant mesothelioma and histopathology (Fig. 3.16u–x) is also shown. Soon after the MRI, about 1.3 years after the right pleural effusion was seen on chest radiograph, the patient expired.

Case 3

A 58-year-old man with a remote smoking history presented with a pulling and pressure sensation deep in the left side of his chest. He has been exposed to various heavy metals from a power plant and possibly has been exposed to asbestos. A chest radiograph (Fig. 3.17a) and PET/CT (Fig. 3.17b, c) were obtained, and a chest CT further characterized the findings (Fig. 3.17d–f). Pleuroscopy was performed (Fig. 3.17g, h) and the diagnosis of malignant mesothelioma was made on a biopsy of the parietal pleura. Later, ultrasonography was obtained for left-sided pleural effusion (Fig. 3.17i, j). A subsequent PET/CT (Fig. 3.17k, l) demonstrated progression of malignant pleural mesothelioma. The patient expired 6 months from the time of the initial chest radiograph.

---

with fissural involvement. No rib erosion is seen. Chest radiographs 6 months later (k, l) show extensive nodular right pleural thickening, multiple bilateral pulmonary nodules, and a new left pleural effusion. MRI of the cervical and thoracic spine was obtained around the same time and axial (m), and coronal (n, o) nonfat-suppressed T2-weighted images demonstrate right pleural masses and nodular thickening of the pleura. Coronal nonfat-suppressed T2-weighted images (p, q) show extension into the endothoracic fascia with involvement of the overlying ribs. There is also fissural pleural nodularity. These pleural masses demonstrate heterogeneous enhancement after the administration of intravenous gadolinium-based contrast agent (r). Pleuroscopic images show diffuse nodular infiltration of the parietal, diaphragmatic, and to a lesser extent, visceral pleura consistent with the diffuse malignant disease (s, t). Biopsies from the right parietal pleura reveal sheets of atypical cells growing in a tumefactive pattern and invading into adipose tissue (u) as also highlighted by an OSCAR keratin immunostain (v). The histologic features are suggestive of a biphasic neoplasm with an epithelioid (w) and a sarcomatoid (x) component. The tumor cells are focally positive for CK5/6, WT-1 and calretinin and lacked staining for TTF-1, napsin, and MOC31 (not shown). The morphologic and immunophenotypical features are consistent with malignant mesothelioma, biphasic type. Magnification × 40 (u, v), × 400 (w, x).(S&T: Courtesy of Dr. Fabien Maldonado, Mayo Clinic Rochester, MN)

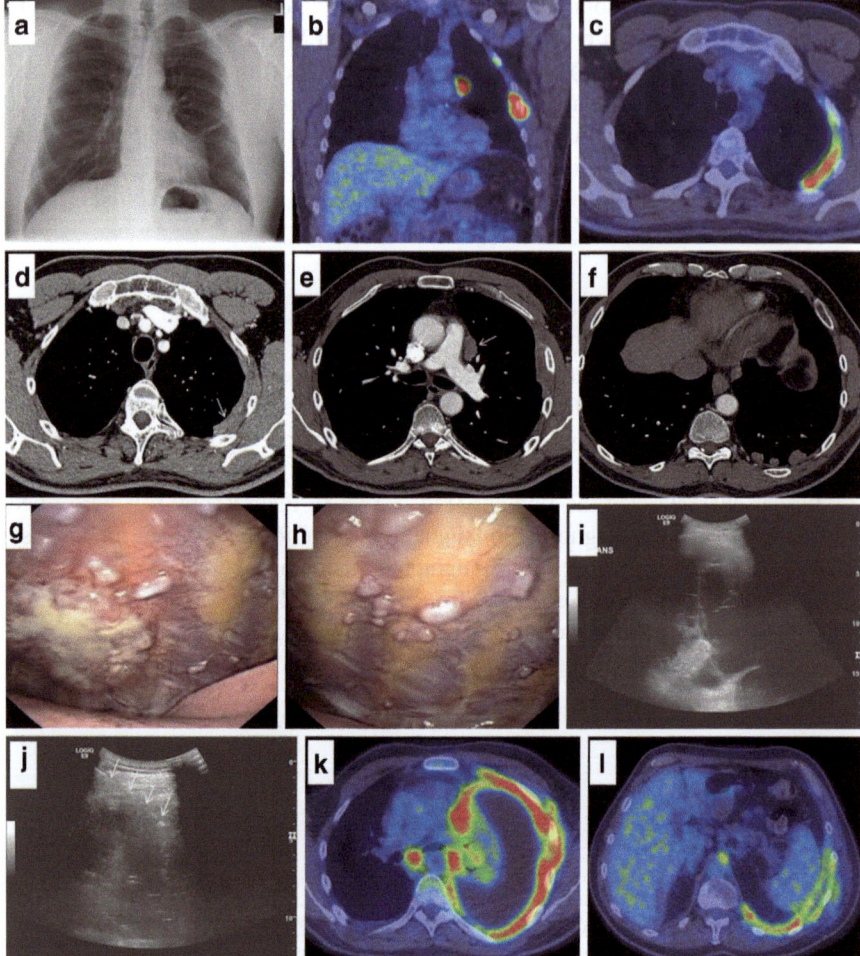

Fig. 3.17 PA chest radiograph (**a**) demonstrats pleural thickening and nodularity about the left lung concerning for metastases or mesothelioma. PET/CT (**b**) shows nodular areas of increased FDG uptake involving the pleura of the left hemithorax both laterally and medially. There are additional areas of hypermetabolic pleural thickening (**c**) on the left. Contrast-enhanced CT of the chest demonstrates plaque-like pleural thickening (*arrow*; **d**), nodules along the mediastinal surface (*arrow*; **e**), and nodules along the left lung base (**f**). Pleuroscopic images (**g, h**) demonstrate areas of dense nodularity consistent with pleural plaque and areas of superimposed soft tissue nodularity consistent with malignancy. Ultrasonography show a moderate to large left pleural effusion with atelectasis of the lung (**i**). An ultrasound-guided thoracentesis (**j**) was performed and the catheter (*arrows*) can be seen traversing thickened pleura. PET/CT (**k, l**) obtained around the same time demonstrate extensive nodular left pleural thickening which has markedly progressed and causes circumferential encasement of the entire left lung. There is also subcarinal lymphadenopathy. (*FDG* fluorodeoxyglucose, *PET/CT* positron emission tomography/computer tomography). (G&H: Courtesy of Dr. Fabien Maldonado, Mayo Clinic Rochester, MN)

References

1. Robinson BW, Musk AW, Lake RA. Malignant mesothelioma. Lancet. 2005;366:397–408.
2. Ismail-Khan R, Robinson LA, Williams CC Jr, Garrett CR, Bepler G, Simon GR. Malignant pleural mesothelioma: a comprehensive review. Cancer Control. 2006;13:255–63.
3. van Meerbeeck JP, Scherpereel A, Surmont VF, Baas P. Malignant pleural mesothelioma: the standard of care and challenges for future management. Crit Rev Oncol Hematol. 2011;78:92–111.
4. Sheard JD, Taylor W, Soorae A, Pearson MG. Pneumothorax and malignant mesothelioma in patients over the age of 40. Thorax. 1991;46:584–5.
5. Alkhuja S, Miller A, Mastellone AJ, Markowitz S. Malignant pleural mesothelioma presenting as spontaneous pneumothorax: a case series and review. Am J Ind Med. 2000;38:219–23.
6. Seely JM, Nguyen ET, Churg AM, Muller NL. Malignant pleural mesothelioma: computed tomography and correlation with histology. Eur J Radiol. 2009;70:485–91.
7. Adams VI, Unni KK, Muhm JR, Jett JR, Ilstrup DM, Bernatz PE. Diffuse malignant mesothelioma of pleura. Diagnosis and survival in 92 cases. Cancer. 1986;58:1540–51.
8. British Thoracic Society Standards of Care Committee. BTS statement on malignant mesothelioma in the UK, 2007. Thorax 2007;62(Suppl 2):ii1–19.
9. Larsen BT, Klein JR, Hornychova H, et al. Diffuse intrapulmonary malignant mesothelioma masquerading as interstitial lung disease: a distinctive variant of mesothelioma. Am J Surg Pathol. 2013;37:1555–64.
10. Rossi G, Cavazza A, Turrini E, et al. Exclusive intrapulmonary lepidic growth of a malignant pleural mesothelioma presenting with pneumothorax and involving the peritoneum. Int J Surg Pathol. 2006;14:234–7.
11. Heki U, Fujimura M, Kasahara K, Matsubara F, Matsuda T. Malignant mesothelioma presenting as pulmonary metastasis ahead of growth of primary tumour. Respirology. 1999;4:279–81.
12. Musk AW, Dewar J, Shilkin KB, Whitaker D. Miliary spread of malignant pleural mesothelioma without a clinically identifiable pleural tumour. Aust NZ J Med. 1991;21:460–2.
13. Nind NR, Attanoos RL, Gibbs AR. Unusual intraparenchymal growth patterns of malignant pleural mesothelioma. Histopathology. 2003;42:150–5.
14. Gunday M, Erinanc H, Geredeli C. Unusual region for pericardial malignant mesothelioma: cutaneous manifestation in a Turkish woman. Rare Tumors. 2013;5:e41.
15. Wild K, Sankaran P, Nagy A, Sington J. Meningeal and brainstem infiltration by a malignant mesothelioma. BMJ Case Rep. 2010.
16. Elbahaie AM, Kamel DE, Lawrence J, Davidson NG. Late cutaneous metastases to the face from malignant pleural mesothelioma: a case report and review of the literature. World J Surg Oncol. 2009;7:84.
17. Sussman J, Rosai J. Lymph node metastasis as the initial manifestation of malignant mesothelioma. Report of six cases. Am J Surg Pathol. 1990;14:819–28.
18. Yakirevich E, Sova Y, Drumea K, Bergman I, Quitt M, Resnick MB. Peripheral lymphadenopathy as the initial manifestation of pericardial mesothelioma: a case report. Int J Surg Pathol. 2004;12:403–5.
19. Craig FE, Fishback NF, Schwartz JG, Powers CN. Occult metastatic mesothelioma–diagnosis by fine-needle aspiration. A case report. Am J Clin Pathol. 1992;97:493–7.
20. Zhang Y, Taheri ZM, Jorda M. Systemic lymphadenopathy as the initial presentation of malignant mesothelioma: a report of three cases. Patholog Res Int. 2010;2010:846571.
21. Lloreta J, Serrano S. Pleural mesothelioma presenting as an axillary lymph node metastasis with anemone cell appearance. Ultrastruct Pathol. 1994;18:293–8.
22. Wills EJ. Pleural mesothelioma with initial presentation as cervical lymphadenopathy. Ultrastruct Pathol. 1995;19:389–94.
23. Tammilehto L, Maasilta P, Kostiainen S, Appelqvist P, Holsti LR, Mattson K. Diagnosis and prognostic factors in malignant pleural mesothelioma: a retrospective analysis of sixty-five patients. Respiration. 1992;59:129–35.

24. Tanrikulu AC, Abakay A, Kaplan MA, et al. A clinical, radiographic and laboratory evaluation of prognostic factors in 363 patients with malignant pleural mesothelioma. Respiration. 2010;80:480–7.
25. Yates DH, Corrin B, Stidolph PN, Browne K. Malignant mesothelioma in south east England: clinicopathological experience of 272 cases. Thorax. 1997;52:507–12.
26. Bani-Hani KE, Gharaibeh KA. Malignant peritoneal mesothelioma. J Surg Oncol. 2005;91:17–25.
27. Bridda A, Padoan I, Mencarelli R, Frego M. Peritoneal mesothelioma: a review. Med Gen Med. 2007;9:32.
28. Eltabbakh GH, Piver MS, Hempling RE, Recio FO, Intengen ME. Clinical picture, response to therapy, and survival of women with diffuse malignant peritoneal mesothelioma. J Surg Oncol. 1999;70:6–12.
29. Asensio JA, Goldblatt P, Thomford NR. Primary malignant peritoneal mesothelioma. A report of seven cases and a review of the literature. Arch Surg. 1990;125:1477–81.
30. Acherman YI, Welch LS, Bromley CM, Sugarbaker PH. Clinical presentation of peritoneal mesothelioma. Tumori. 2003;89:269–73.
31. Ribak J, Lilis R, Suzuki Y, Penner L, Selikoff IJ. Malignant mesothelioma in a cohort of asbestos insulation workers: clinical presentation, diagnosis, and causes of death. Br J Ind Med. 1988;45:182–7.
32. Salemis NS, Tsiambas E, Gourgiotis S, Mela A, Karameris A, Tsohataridis E. Peritoneal mesothelioma presenting as an acute surgical abdomen due to jejunal perforation. J Dig Dis. 2007;8:216–21.
33. Yan TD, Popa E, Brun EA, Cerruto CA, Sugarbaker PH. Sex difference in diffuse malignant peritoneal mesothelioma. Br J Surg. 2006;93:1536–42.
34. Mani H, Merino MJ. Mesothelial neoplasms presenting as, and mimicking, ovarian cancer. Int J Gynecol Pathol. 2010;29:523–8.
35. Baker PM, Clement PB, Young RH. Malignant peritoneal mesothelioma in women: a study of 75 cases with emphasis on their morphologic spectrum and differential diagnosis. Am J Clin Pathol. 2005;123:724–37.
36. Manzini VP, Recchia L, Cafferata M, et al. Malignant peritoneal mesothelioma: a multicenter study on 81 cases. Ann Oncol. 2010;21:348–53.
37. Schneiderman H. Mesothelioma and venous thrombosis. CMAJ. 2004;171:11, author reply -2.
38. Banayan S, Hot A, Janier M, Ninet J, Zurlinden O, Billotey C. Malignant mesothelioma of the peritoneum as the cause of a paraneoplastic syndrome: detection by 18F-FDG PET. Eur J Nucl Med Mol Imaging. 2006;33:751.
39. Socola F, Loaiza-Bonilla A, Bustinza-Linares E, Correa R, Rosenblatt JD. Recurrent thrombotic thrombocytopenic purpura-like syndrome as a paraneoplastic phenomenon in malignant peritoneal mesothelioma: a case report and review of the literature. Case Rep Oncol Med. 2012;2012:619348.
40. Bech C, Sorensen JB. Polyneuropathy in a patient with malignant pleural mesothelioma: a paraneoplastic syndrome. J Thorac Oncol. 2008;3:1359–60.
41. Archer HA, Panopoulou A, Bhatt N, Edey AJ, Giffin NJ. Mesothelioma and anti-Ma paraneoplastic syndrome; heterogeneity in immunogenic tumours increases. Pract Neurol. 2014;14(1):33–5.
42. Tanriverdi O, Meydan N, Barutca S, Ozsan N, Gurel D, Veral A. Anti-Yo antibody-mediated paraneoplastic cerebellar degeneration in a female patient with pleural malignant mesothelioma. Jpn J Clin Oncol. 2013;43:563–8.
43. Britton M. The epidemiology of mesothelioma. Semin Oncol. 2002;29:18–25.
44. Jarvholm B, Sanden A. Lung cancer and mesothelioma in the pleura and peritoneum among Swedish insulation workers. Occup Environ Med. 1998;55:766–70.
45. Hilliard AK, Lovett JK, McGavin CR. The rise and fall in incidence of malignant mesothelioma from a British Naval Dockyard, 1979–1999. Occup Med (Lond). 2003;53:209–12.

46. Abakay A, Tanrikulu AC, Kaplan MA, et al. Clinical characteristics and treatment outcomes in 132 patients with malignant mesothelioma. Lung India. 2011;28:267–71.
47. Antman KH, Blum RH, Greenberger JS, Flowerdew G, Skarin AT, Canellos GP. Multimodality therapy for malignant mesothelioma based on a study of natural history. Am J Med. 1980;68:356–62.
48. Rosas-Salazar C, Gunawardena SW, Spahr JE. Malignant pleural mesothelioma in a child with ataxia-telangiectasia. Pediatr Pulmonol. 2013;48:94–7.
49. Fraire AE, Cooper S, Greenberg SD, Buffler P, Langston C. Mesothelioma of childhood. Cancer. 1988;62:838–47.
50. Moran CA, Albores-Saavedra J, Suster S. Primary peritoneal mesotheliomas in children: a clinicopathological and immunohistochemical study of eight cases. Histopathology. 2008;52:824–30.
51. Light RW, Macgregor MI, Luchsinger PC, Ball WC Jr. Pleural effusions: the diagnostic separation of transudates and exudates. Ann Intern Med. 1972;77:507–13.
52. Gottehrer A, Taryle DA, Reed CE, Sahn SA. Pleural fluid analysis in malignant mesothelioma. Prognostic implications. Chest. 1991;100:1003–6.
53. Pass HI, Levin SM, Harbut MR, et al. Fibulin-3 as a blood and effusion biomarker for pleural mesothelioma. N Engl J Med. 2012;367:1417–27.
54. Campbell NP, Kindler HL. Update on malignant pleural mesothelioma. Semin Respir Crit Care Med. 2011;32:102–10.
55. Pass HI, Lott D, Lonardo F, et al. Asbestos exposure, pleural mesothelioma, and serum osteopontin levels. N Engl J Med. 2005;353:1564–73.
56. Shi HZ, Liang QL, Jiang J, Qin XJ, Yang HB. Diagnostic value of carcinoembryonic antigen in malignant pleural effusion: a meta-analysis. Respirology. 2008;13:518–27.
57. Grigoriu BD, Grigoriu C, Chahine B, Gey T, Scherpereel A. Clinical utility of diagnostic markers for malignant pleural mesothelioma. Monaldi Arch Chest Dis. 2009;71:31–8.
58. Fuhrman C, Duche JC, Chouaid C, et al. Use of tumor markers for differential diagnosis of mesothelioma and secondary pleural malignancies. Clin Biochem. 2000;33:405–10.
59. Frebourg T, Lerebours G, Delpech B, et al. Serum hyaluronate in malignant pleural mesothelioma. Cancer. 1987;59:2104–7.
60. Chiu B, Churg A, Tengblad A, Pearce R, McCaughey WT. Analysis of hyaluronic acid in the diagnosis of malignant mesothelioma. Cancer. 1984;54:2195–9.
61. Creaney J, Dick IM, Segal A, Musk AW, Robinson BW. Pleural effusion hyaluronic acid as a prognostic marker in pleural malignant mesothelioma. Lung Cancer. 2013;82:491–8.
62. Filiberti R, Parodi S, Libener R, et al. Diagnostic value of mesothelin in pleural fluids: comparison with CYFRA 21-1 and CEA. Med Oncol. 2013;30:543.
63. O'Rahilly R, Muller NL, Carpenter S, Swenson R. Basic human anatomy: A regional study of human structure. Chapter 22. In: O'Rahilly R, editor. Online version. Dartmouth Medical School and Dartmouth College, New Hampshire, USA; 2008.
64. Gray H, editor. Anatomy of the human body. New York: Bartleby.com; 2000.
65. Rusch VW. A proposed new international TNM staging system for malignant pleural mesothelioma from the International Mesothelioma Interest Group. Lung Cancer. 1996;14:1–12.
66. Rusch VW, Giroux D. Do we need a revised staging system for malignant pleural mesothelioma? Analysis of the IASLC database. Ann Cardiothorac Surg. 2012;1:438–48.
67. Rusch VW, Giroux D, Kennedy C, et al. Initial analysis of the international association for the study of lung cancer mesothelioma database. J Thorac Oncol. 2012;7:1631–9.
68. Kawashima A, Libshitz HI. Malignant pleural mesothelioma: CT manifestations in 50 cases. AJR Am J Roentgenol. 1990;155:965–9.
69. Metintas M, Ucgun I, Elbek O, et al. Computed tomography features in malignant pleural mesothelioma and other commonly seen pleural diseases. Eur J Radiol. 2002;41:1–9.
70. Armato SG 3rd, Labby ZE, Coolen J, et al. Imaging in pleural mesothelioma: a review of the 11th International Conference of the International Mesothelioma Interest Group. Lung Cancer. 2013;82:190–6.

71. Corson N, Sensakovic WF, Straus C, Starkey A, Armato SG 3rd. Characterization of mesothelioma and tissues present in contrast-enhanced thoracic CT scans. Med Phys. 2011;38:942–7.
72. Patz EF Jr, Shaffer K, Piwnica-Worms DR, et al. Malignant pleural mesothelioma: value of CT and MR imaging in predicting resectability. AJR Am J Roentgenol. 1992;159:961–6.
73. Heelan RT, Rusch VW, Begg CB, Panicek DM, Caravelli JF, Eisen C. Staging of malignant pleural mesothelioma: comparison of CT and MR imaging. AJR Am J Roentgenol. 1999;172:1039–47.
74. Coolen J, De Keyzer F, Nafteux P, et al. Malignant pleural disease: diagnosis by using diffusion-weighted and dynamic contrast-enhanced MR imaging–initial experience. Radiology. 2012;263:884–92.
75. Byrne MJ, Nowak AK. Modified RECIST criteria for assessment of response in malignant pleural mesothelioma. Ann Oncol. 2004;15:257–60.
76. Sensakovic WF, Armato SG 3rd, Starkey A, Kindler HL, Vigneswaran WT. Quantitative measurement of lung reexpansion in malignant pleural mesothelioma patients undergoing pleurectomy/decortication. Acad Radiol. 2011;18:294–8.
77. Flores RM. The role of PET in the surgical management of malignant pleural mesothelioma. Lung Cancer. 2005;49(Suppl 1):S27–32.
78. Flores RM, Akhurst T, Gonen M, Larson SM, Rusch VW. Positron emission tomography defines metastatic disease but not locoregional disease in patients with malignant pleural mesothelioma. J Thorac Cardiovasc Surg. 2003;126:11–6.
79. Truong MT, Viswanathan C, Godoy MB, Carter BW, Marom EM. Malignant pleural mesothelioma: role of CT, MRI, and PET/CT in staging evaluation and treatment considerations. Semin Roentgenol. 2013;48:323–34.
80. Duysinx B, Nguyen D, Louis R, et al. Evaluation of pleural disease with 18-fluorodeoxyglucose positron emission tomography imaging. Chest. 2004;125:489–93.
81. Kinahan PE, Fletcher JW. Positron emission tomography-computed tomography standardized uptake values in clinical practice and assessing response to therapy. Semin Ultrasound CT MR. 2010;31:496–505.
82. Margolis DJ, Hoffman JM, Herfkens RJ, Jeffrey RB, Quon A, Gambhir SS. Molecular imaging techniques in body imaging. Radiology. 2007;245:333–56.
83. Jeon KN, Bae K, Park MJ, et al. US-guided transthoracic biopsy of peripheral lung lesions: pleural contact length influences diagnostic yield. Acta Radiol. 2014;55(3):295–301.
84. Yang PC. Ultrasound-guided transthoracic biopsy of peripheral lung, pleural, and chest-wall lesions. J Thorac Imaging. 1997;12:272–84.
85. Law MR, Hodson ME, Turner-Warwick M. Malignant mesothelioma of the pleura: clinical aspects and symptomatic treatment. Eur J Respir Dis. 1984;65:162–8.

Chapter 4
Histology

Mahmoud Eltorky

Introduction

Diffuse malignant mesothelioma (DMM) is a relatively rare but unique neoplasm of the pleura and other serosal surfaces. In the last half century, DMM has been the subject of numerous epidemiologic, clinical, experimental, and pathologic studies. Enormous medical and legal interest has been generated by rising DMM incidence, particularly after the recognition of asbestos as a causative agent [1, 2, 3]. DMM diagnosis can be accomplished at several levels during the pathologic evaluation, beginning with gross and microscopic examination and extending through immunohistochemical, molecular, and occasionally even electron microscopic confirmation.

Gross and Microscopic Features

The gross features of DMM are often of paramount importance in rendering accurate diagnoses. Pleural DMM is more common on the right than on the left, in a ratio of 3:2 [1]. Early stages of pleural involvement by mesothelioma usually consist of parietal pleural involvement by small numerous nodules. Visceral pleura less frequently may develop similar features as well [4, 5]. Subsequent growth of the neoplastic nodules leads to its coalescence; overtime progression of the lesion occurs with extensive involvement of the pleural surface resulting in fusion of visceral and parietal pleura with encasement and contraction of the lung (Fig. 4.1). Tumor growth follows the distribution on the pleural surface. The circumferential rind of tumor at late stage is typically lobulated, firm, and white (Fig. 4.2). The tumor tracks along the pleural reflections into the lung fissures with a finger-like extension

---

M. Eltorky (✉)
Department of Pathology, University of Texas Medical Branch,
301 University Blvd., Galveston, TX 77555, USA
e-mail: maeltork@utmb.edu

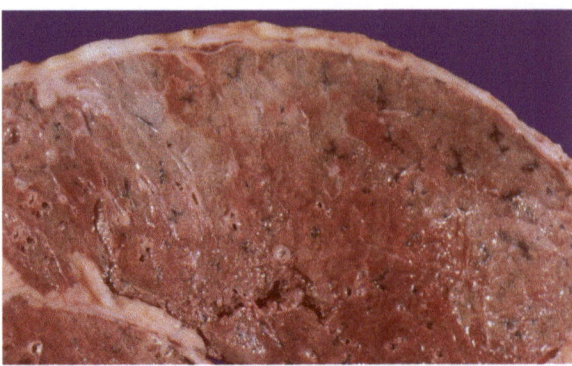

Fig. 4.1 Diffuse malignant mesothelioma: The tumor completely encases the lung and extends along the fissure

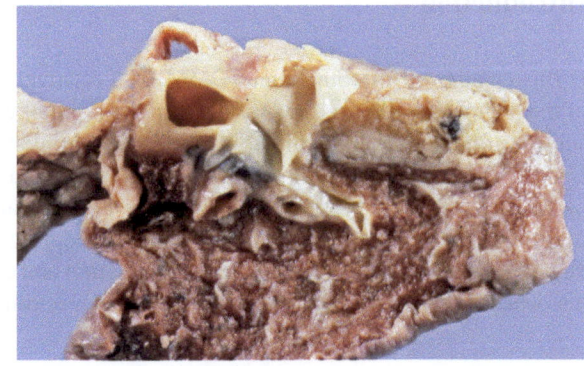

Fig. 4.2 Diffuse malignant mesothelioma: The tumor at the *lower right* corner envelop the lung and on the *upper* field encases the bronchvascular bundle and invade the lung

into interlobular septa and underlying lung. The tumor may reach several centimeters in thickness and range from firm to gelatinous in consistency. Mediastinal involvement with invasion of the pericardium, chest wall fat, and muscle involvement is characteristic. Pleural DMM may grow along needle tracts or biopsy incisions, and then manifest as a subcutaneous tumor nodule [6]. Metastases to mediastinal and hilar lymph nodes and lungs are usually evident of advanced-stage disease.

Microscopically, DMM features a wide range of histopathologic variants. The World Health Organization [7] recognizes three broad basic histologic variants of DMM: epithelial, sarcomatous, and biphasic.

Epithelial Diffuse Malignant Mesothelioma

Epithelial DMM is the most common histologic variant [7], a wide range of morphologic patterns are seen. The most frequent patterns are tubulopapillary, the solid patterns [8, 9, 10], and adenomatoid (microglandular). Sometimes, one pattern predominates but several different patterns are commonly seen in the same tumor. Less common patterns include small cell, clear cell, and deciduoid. Most epithelial

Fig. 4.3 Epithelial malignant mesothelioma showing cuboidal cells with moderate amount of eosinophilic cytoplasm with bland relatively open nuclei and infrequent mitosis

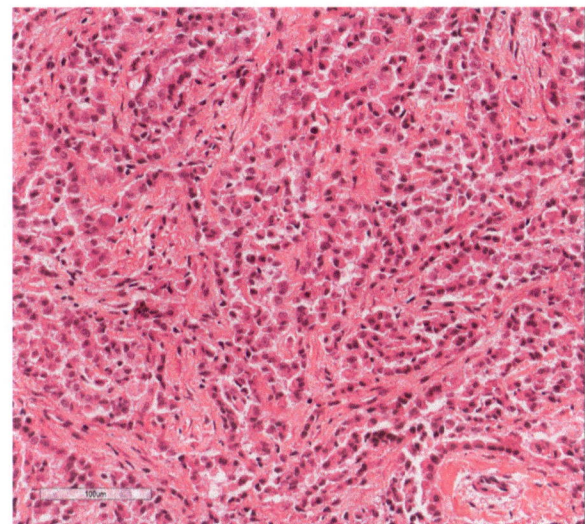

Fig. 4.4 High-grade (pleomorphic) epithelial mesothelioma showing prominent nucleoli with frequent mitosis and considerable cell-to-cell variation

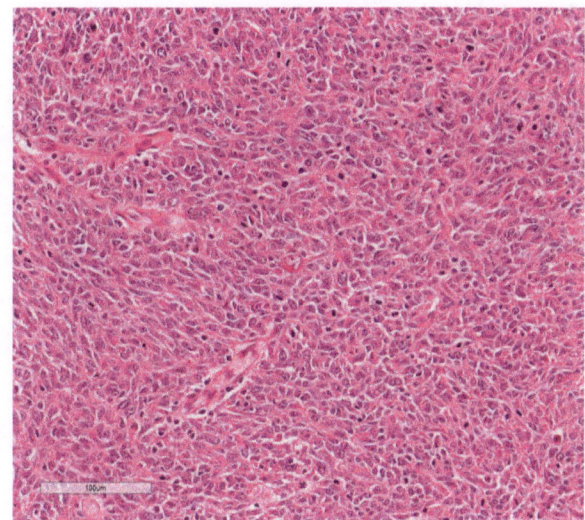

DMM is cytologically monotonous and remarkably bland in appearance. The tumor cells are typically cuboidal with moderate amount of eosinophilic cytoplasm with bland and relatively open nuclei and infrequent mitosis (Fig. 4.3). In the less differentiated area, the nuclei show coarse chromatin and prominent nucleoli with frequent mitosis and considerable cell-to-cell variation of such tumor when that pattern predominate the term high-grade (pleomorphic) epithelial DMM will apply (Fig. 4.4). Such tumor is difficult to distinguish from metastatic carcinoma based on routine hematoxylin–eosin (H&E) histology alone.

Fig. 4.5 Epithelial mesothelioma showing tubulopapillary pattern with outwards secondary branching

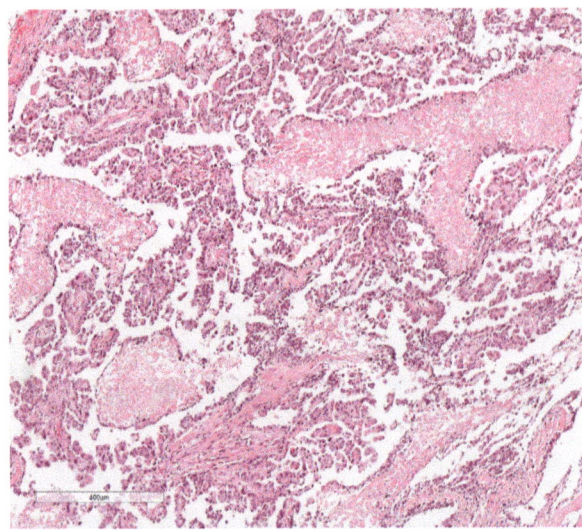

Fig. 4.6 Epithelial mesothelioma with tubopapillary pattern shows the glands and the papillae are covered by single layer of cuboidal to flattened cells

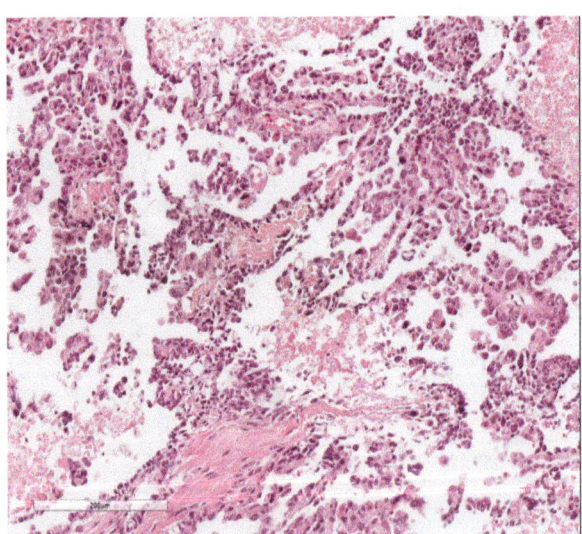

The most frequent pattern is often referred to as tubulopapillary (Fig. 4.5). In this pattern, the glands and the papillae are covered by a single layer of cuboidal to flattened cells (Fig. 4.6). Psammoma bodies may be seen but are usually infrequent [11].

Epithelial DMM may show microcytic (adenomatoid; Fig. 4.7) pattern which is usually composed of flattened bland-looking mesothelial cells; careful examination reveals the presence of some cells with large nuclei and prominent nucleoli and the tumor cells show infiltrative and diffuse pattern [12]. Further examination reveals areas of transition to ordinary patterns of epithelial DMM.

Fig. 4.7 Epithelial mesotheliomas with infiltrative microcytic (adenomatoid) pattern composed of flattened bland looking mesothelial cells

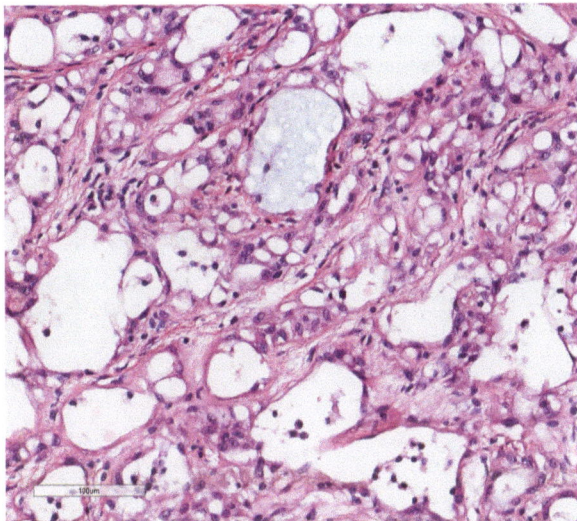

Fig. 4.8 Epithelial mesothelioma with solid infiltrative pattern

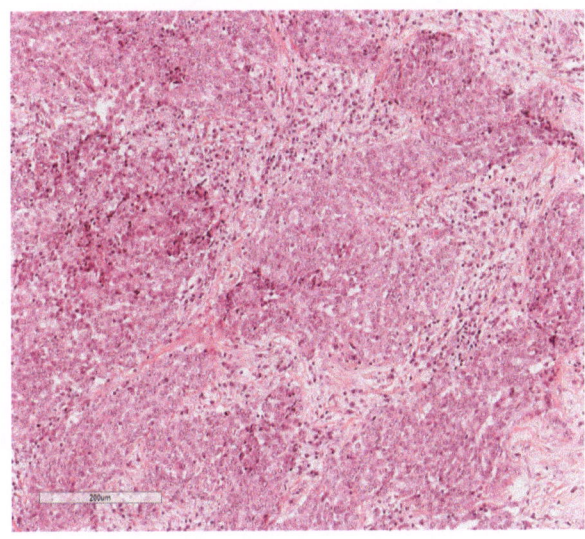

Epithelial DMM may also exhibit a predominantly solid sheet-like pattern (Fig. 4.8). In this pattern, the malignant cells form solid sheets of epithelioid cells with abundant eosinophilic cytoplasm with vesicular nuclei and prominent nucleoli; the tumor cells may contain cytoplasmic vacuoles mimicking signet ring carcinoma (Fig. 4.9). The vacuoles are rich in hyaluronate which stain strongly with Alcian blue, pH 2.5, and digested by prior hyalurinidase treatment [13].

The extremely rare small cell pattern [14, 15] of epithelial DMM is composed of fairly small cells mimicking small cell carcinoma of the lung. The mesothelial cells are arranged in monotonous sheets with no crush artifacts or basophilic staining of

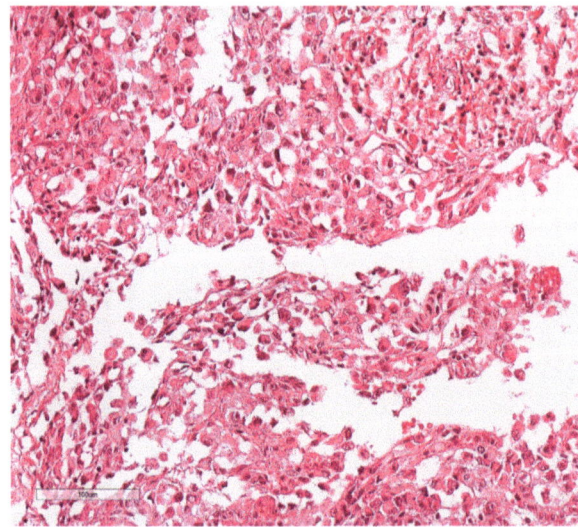

Fig. 4.9 Epithelial mesothelioma showing polygonal cells with dense eosinophilic cytoplasm and some cells with cytoplasmic vacuoles

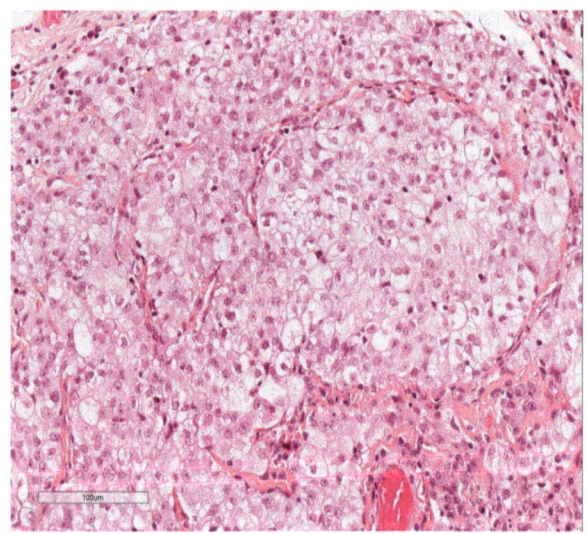

Fig. 4.10 Epithelial mesothelioma with clear cell type, this pattern must be differentiated from metastatic renal cell carcinoma

blood vessels wall. Furthermore, the nuclear chromatin is open with low mitosis. The neuroendocrine markers are usually negative. Further examination of the submitted tissue shows transition to typical patterns of epithelial DMM.

The clear cell [16] pattern shows a loosely arranged sheet of clear cells. Further examination of the tumor reveals areas of transition to more typical DMM patterns. Occasionally, clear tumor cells predominate (Fig. 4.10), and the tumor must be distinguished from metastatic renal cell carcinoma. Immunohistochemical and, if necessary, ultrastructure examination will confirm the mesothelial nature of the neoplastic cells.

Fig. 4.11 Epithelial mesothelioma. The tumor show some cells with deciduoid pattern with large cells that resemble decidua

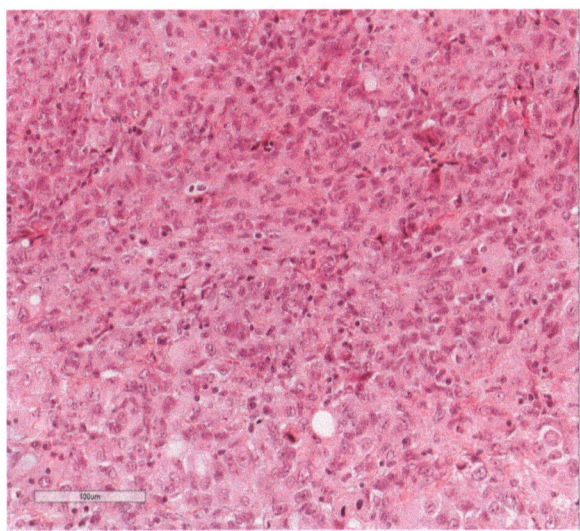

The deciduoid pattern [17–19] consists of large polygonal cells with abundant eosinophilic cytoplasm similar to decidual cells (Fig. 4.11). Sometimes, there is transition from deciduoid form to other typical mesothelial patterns. Immunohistochemistry will confirm the mesothelial origin of the tumor cells.

Sarcomatous Diffuse Malignant Mesothelioma

Sarcomatous DMM is an aggressive type of malignant mesothelioma which histologically exhibits a wide range of architectural complexity from hypocellular collections of extremely bland spindle cells to densely cellular areas with obviously high-grade cellular features. The most common pattern consists of closely packed bland-looking spindled cells arranged in fascicles resembling fibrosarcoma (Fig. 4.12) or obviously malignant spindle cells with multinucleated giant cells and a storiform pattern, resembling so-called malignant fibrous histiocytoma (Fig. 4.13). A combination of different patterns may be seen in the same tumor [20–22].

The spindle cells of sarcomatous DMM range from bland spindle cells with a long and thin cytoplasm (Fig. 4.14) to marked anaplasia with bizarre nuclei and increased mitotic figures as shown in Fig. 4.13. In small percentage of cases heterologous elements in the form of malignant cartilage, bone, smooth or skeletal muscles occur, mimicking chondrosarcoma, osteosarcoma, leiomyosarcoma, or rhabdomyosarcoma [3, 23–25]. All these are referred to as sarcomatous DMM. Differentiation of sarcomatoid DMM with heterologous elements from primary sarcoma of pleura may be accomplished by focal or diffuse immunohistochemical staining for broad-spectrum cytokeratin (CK) 5/6 and calretinin or ultrastructure examination. There are two additional morphologic variants of sarcomatoid DMM: lymphohistiocytoid variant of sarcomatoid DMM and desmoplastic DMM.

Fig. 4.12 Sarcomatous mesothelioma showing malignant spindle cells with arranged in fascicles resemble fibrosarcoma

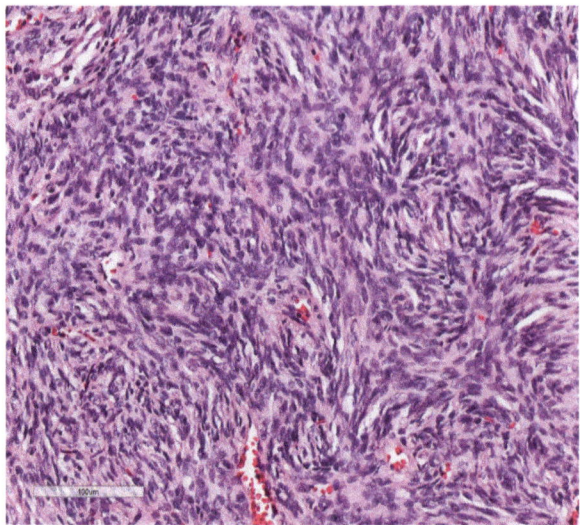

Fig. 4.13 A sarcomatous mesothelioma showing the storiform pattern and the high grade nuclei and occasional multinucleated giant cells a typical features seen in sarcomatous mesothelioma

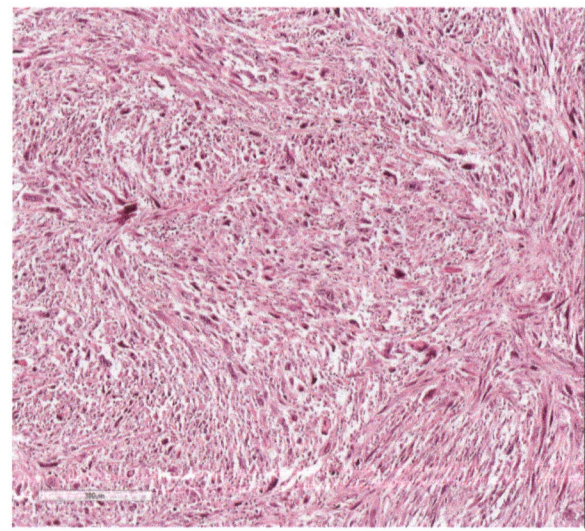

The lymphohistiocytoid variant was first described by Henderson in 1988. [26] This variant of sarcomatoid DMM is characterized by intense chronic inflammatory cell infiltrate of small lymphocytes, plasma cells, and on occasion, eosinophils intermixed with large polygonal to spindle malignant cells with vesicular nuclei and prominent nucleoli (Figs. 4.15 and 4.16). The malignant cells are positive with (CK)5/6 and Calretinin and negative with lymphoma markers. It is important to recognize this variant due to it similarity to malignant lymphoma [27]. The survival of this neoplasm is similar to those of epithelial DMM.

Fig. 4.14 Sarcomatous mesothelioma showing infiltrative relatively bland looking spindle cells with a long and thin cytoplasm

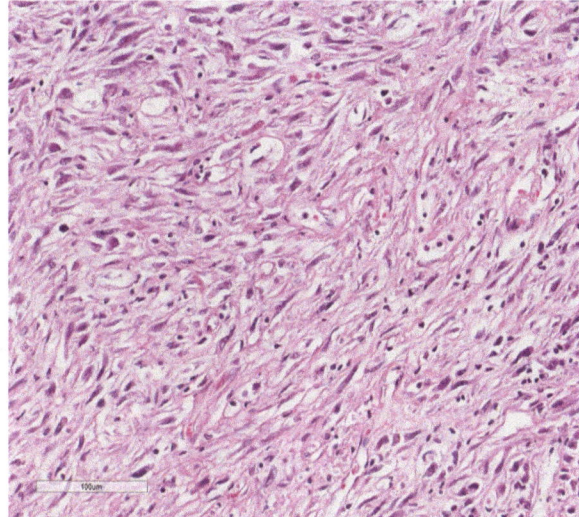

Fig. 4.15 Lymphoepithelioid mesothelioma. The tumor may resemble large cell lymphoma

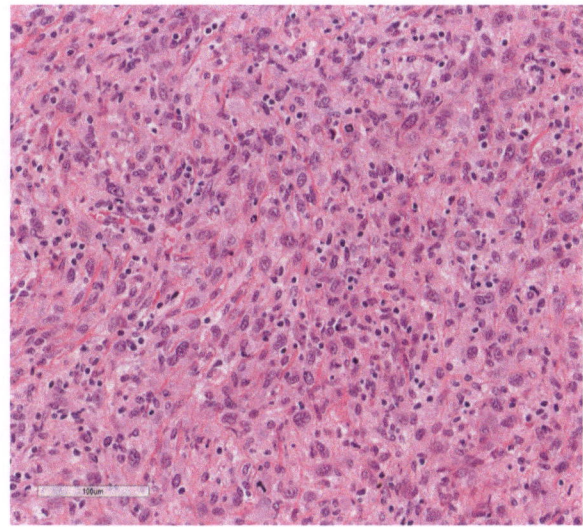

Desmoplastic DMM is a rare and extremely aggressive variant of sarcomatous DMM [28–30]. This subtype, accounting for approximately 5–10% of DMM, was first described by Kannerstein and Churg in 1980 [31]. Histopathologic evaluation shows a dense paucicellular hyalinized collagen among which spindle or stellate tumor cells, often associated with slit-like spaces (Fig. 4.17), are arranged in a storiform or patternless arrangement. Sarcomatous foci are usually present and epithelioid foci can occasionally be seen. Diagnosis of DMM requires the identification of characteristic paucicellular, densely collagenous tissue in addition to the presence of frankly sarcomatous areas (Fig. 4.18), in conjunction with one or more of the following features that are considered highly specific for DMM:

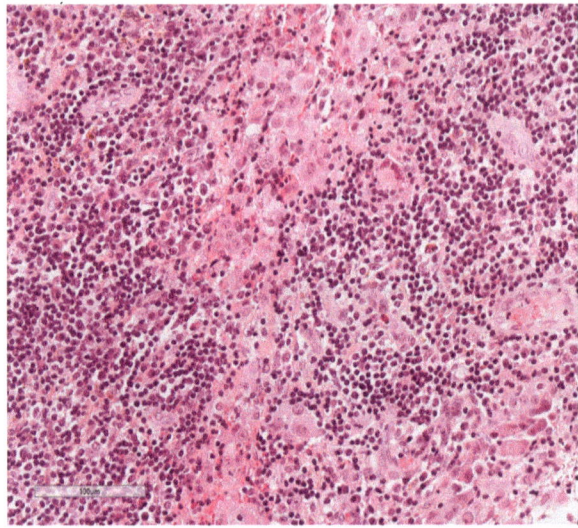

Fig. 4.16 Lymphoepithelioid mesothelioma. High-power view of the histiocytoid tumor cells intermixed with lymphocytes, a feature which may resemble large cell lymphoma

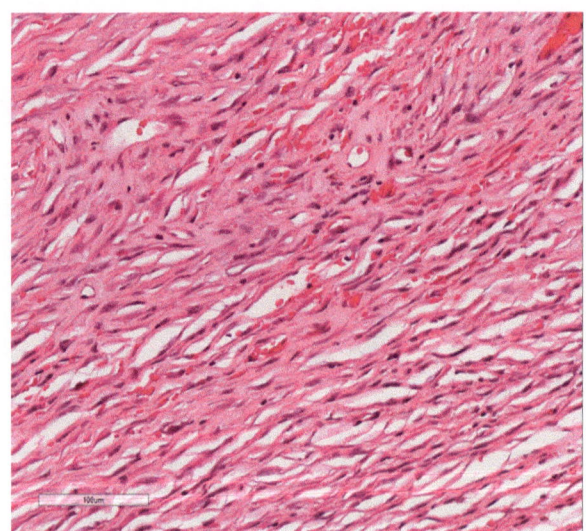

Fig. 4.17 Desmoplastic mesotheliomas. High-power view shows the patterns pattern with a dense paucicellular hyalinized collagen among which spindle or stellate tumor cells

1. Bland infarct-like (no cellular debris or karyorrhexis) sharply demarcated necrosis (Fig. 4.19).
2. Invasion of the chest wall adipose tissue or muscle or the lung (Fig. 4.20).
3. Presence of expansile nodules, (Fig. 4.21).
4. Distant metastasis.

The presence of these features assists in distinguishing desmoplastic DMM from reactive fibrous pleuritis. Infiltration of the underlying chest wall adipose tissue, with isolation of individual adipocytes (Fig. 4.20), is typically confirmed with keratin immunostain. [32, 33].

Fig. 4.18 Desmoplastic mesothelioma low-power view showing characteristic paucicellular, densely collagenous tissue upper field in addition to the presence of frankly sarcomatous areas in the lower field

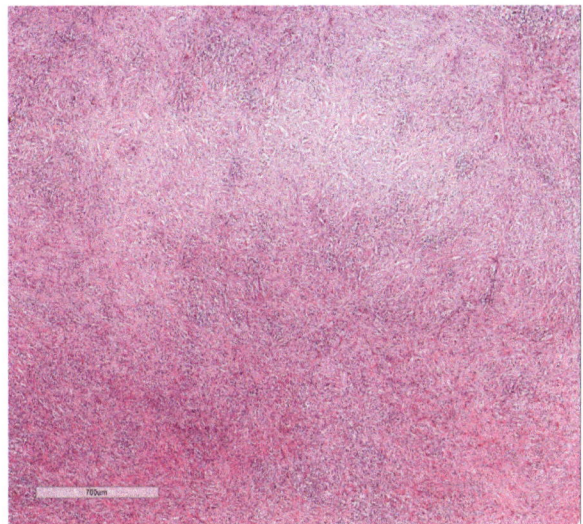

Fig. 4.19 Desmoplastic mesothelioma showing area of bland necrosis in the *lower left* corner

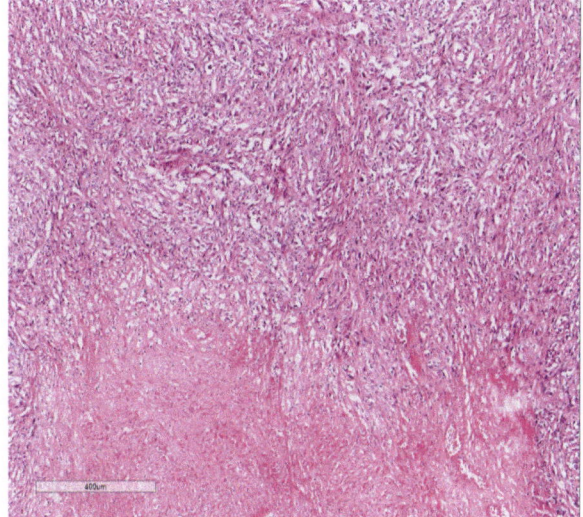

Biphasic Diffuse Malignant Mesothelioma

Approximately 20–35 % of DMM are classified as biphasic DMM. This type is frequently identified in pleural DMM patients. Any combination of epithelial or sarcomatous pattern may be present (Fig. 4.22). According to WHO [7], each component must represent at least 10 % of the tumor to meet the criteria for the diagnosis of biphasic DMM.

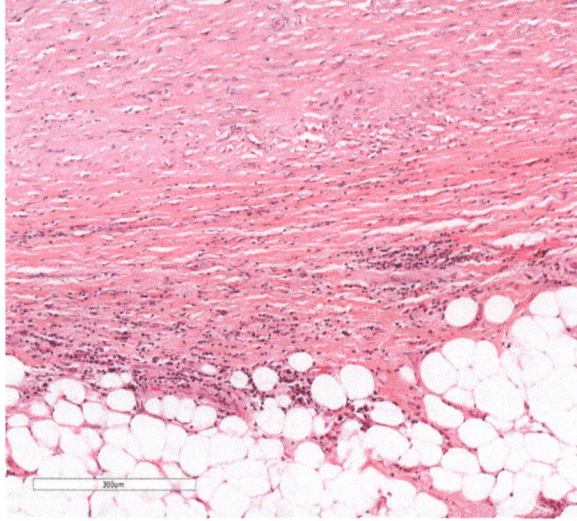

Fig. 4.20 Desmoplastic mesothelioma showing invasion of the chest wall adipose tissue, a feature not seen in fibrosing pleuritis

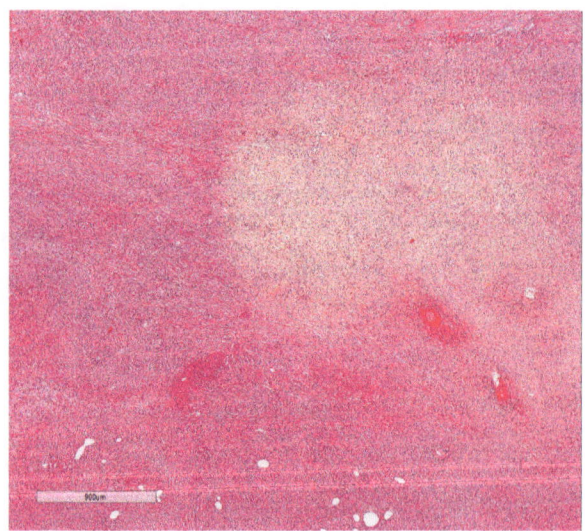

Fig. 4.21 Desmoplastic mesothelioma showing presence of expansile nodule in the *upper right*

Differential Diagnosis of Diffuse Malignant Mesothelioma

The differential diagnosis of DMM includes pleural diffuse or localized neoplastic or nonneoplastic (inflammatory/reactive/infectious) processes. The distinction between these entities almost always requires the correlation of clinical, radiographic, gross, microscopic, and immunohistochemical studies. Some differential diagnoses are common and important to discuss.

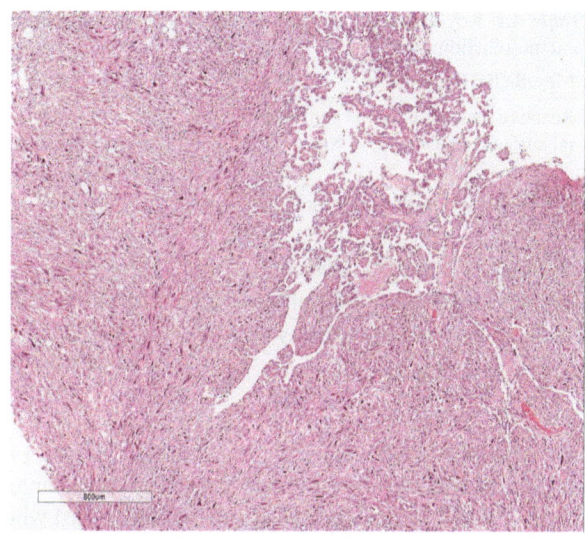

Fig. 4.22 Biphasic malignant mesothelioma showing an area (*upper right*) of epithelial and area (*Left*) of sarcomatous mesothelioma in the same tumor

Epithelial Diffuse Malignant Mesothelioma and Adenocarcinoma

The differential diagnosis between epithelial DMM and lung adenocarcinoma is a well-known diagnostic challenge in surgical pathology, and it is of critical importance for proper medical management. It is also of major importance for legal proceedings that frequently accompany a proposed DMM diagnosis. Both diseases may involve the pleural surfaces and, in most instances, their overlapping histological features preclude a definitive diagnosis based on conventional light microscopic examination. Several ancillary diagnostic techniques, particularly immunohistochemistry, have been employed to assist in rendering accurate diagnoses in these situations [34–36]. The diagnostic utility of conventional histochemical stains alone is limited. Lung adenocarcinomas are not consistently positive for intracytoplasmic mucicarmine and PAS after diastase digestion. Furthermore, false positivity may be observed in a few epithelioid DMM due to technical reasons [14]. The alcian blue-positive, hyalurinidase-sensitive reaction has also been reported in lung adenocarcinomas [15]. Electron microscopy has proven to be useful and is often considered as the gold standard in the diagnosis of epithelial mesothelioma [37, 38]; however, electron microscopic study generally requires great expense and time compared with the other diagnostic techniques, and the morphological ultrastructural features of mesothelial differentiation may not be apparent in the less-differentiated tumors. Furthermore, it may be difficult to obtain. Immunohistochemistry is a generally reliable and typically utilized tool in differentiating DMM from other lesions.

The International Mesothelioma Panel [39] recommends that, at a minimum, two mesothelial and two carcinoma immunomarkers can be used in addition to a pancytokeratin immunostain in rendering a diagnosis. None of these antibodies are 100 % specific and false positives (which often show less than 10 % staining) can occur in

Table 4.1 Key histologic features in differentiation between reactive mesothelial proliferation and mesothelioma

Mesothelial hyperplasia	Mesothelioma
Reactive mesothelial cells confined to pleural surface (superficial)	Nests of mesothelial cells in and surrounded by stroma or papillary pattern with secondary or tertiary branching
Entrapped uniform linear mesothelial nests	Irregular nests of invasive mesothelial cells in underlining stroma
Abundant inflammatory cells	Minimal inflammatory response
Necrosis if present is usually inflammatory	Bland tumor necrosis usually present
No invasion of underlying tissues	Invasion of chest wall fat or muscle, or invasion of lung parenchyma

any neoplasm. Positive thyroid transcription factor 1 (TTF-1) is considered a valuable immunostain for diagnosing lung adenocarcinoma. DMM are immunonegative with TTF-1. The diagnosis is most straightforward when only DMM or carcinoma markers are positive, but in some cases the staining results are conflicting or ambiguous. In those cases, it is often useful to expand the staining panel to include additional markers. If the result continues to be conflicting, electron microscopy may be considered to assist in accurate diagnosis.

Primary adenocarcinomas in other organs—including tumors from the breast, kidney, and ovary, thyroid, pancreas, and kidney—often metastasize to the pleura. Most breast carcinomas will express estrogen receptor, progesterone receptor, and/or mammaglobin. Ovarian serous carcinoma will stain for WT-1, ER, and PR.

Epithelial Diffuse Malignant Mesothelioma and Reactive Mesothelial Cell Hyperplasia

Reactive mesothelial cell hyperplasia may mimic DMM or metastatic carcinoma. Some of the causes of reactive mesothelial cell hyperplasia in the pleural space include infections, pulmonary infarcts, drug reactions, pneumothorax, collagen vascular diseases, lung carcinomas, surgery, trauma, and nonspecific inflammation.

The cytologic features of a reactive mesothelial proliferation that may mimic a neoplasm include high cellularity, the presence of numerous mitotic figures and cytologic atypia, the presence of inflammatory type of necrosis, the formation of papillary groups, and entrapment of reactive mesothelial cells within fibrous tissue of pleural biopsy mimicking invasion [39–42]. Features distinguishing reactive mesothelial hyperplasia from DMM are summarized in Table 4.1.

Stromal or fat invasion is considered an important feature in the diagnosis of DMM (Fig. 4.20). Invasion may involve the visceral and/or parietal pleura and may extend to other adjacent structures; the extent of invasion can be highlighted by pancytokeratin or calretinin immunostain. Invasive mesothelial cells may appear deceptively bland, completely lack a desmoplastic reaction, and involve only a few

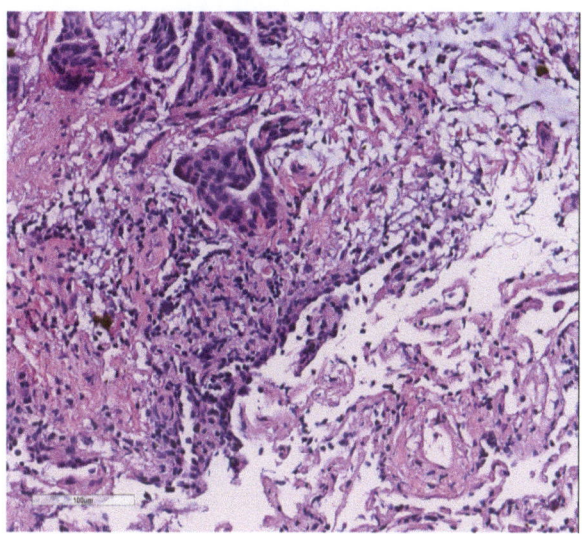

Fig. 4.23 Epithelial mesothelioma. Showing a deep area of the tumor that invades the lung parenchyma, right lower corner

layers of submesothelial collagenous tissue. However, identification of invasion is not absolutely necessary for the diagnosis of DMM. For example, in cases where there is a large solid piece of malignant tumor with histologic features of DMM, invasion may not be absolutely required for diagnosis [39].

Invasion of the fat, muscle, or lung parenchyma continues to be by far the most reliable criterion for separating benign from malignant mesothelial proliferations. Fat is the stroma most frequently encountered and the finding of mesothelial cells growing between fat cells is a strong evidence of the malignant mesothelial cell proliferation unless there is an extraordinarily good reason to believe otherwise. The same comment applies to invasion of muscle or invasion of lung (Fig. 4.23) or distant metastasis. Pankeratin stains are extremely helpful in showing the distribution of mesothelial cells. They are particularly valuable for detecting subtle invasion of fat by a few cells that may not be readily apparent on H&E staining.

Reactive mesothelial proliferations tend to show uniformity of growth with linear arrangements of mesothelial cells, tubules, or small nests (Fig. 4.24), and this uniformity may be confirmed with pancytokeratin immunostain, which will highlight the regular sheets and fascicles of mesothelial cells that respect mesothelial boundaries in contrast to the irregular disorganized growth of DMM.

Mesothelial cell proliferations that are confined to the surface can be benign or malignant; proliferations that reach from the free surface of the thickened pleura to invade the fat or forming papillary architecture with secondary or tertiary branching are almost always malignant (Figs. 4.20 and 4.5). Linear arrangements of mesothelial cells or simple gland-like structures arrayed parallel to the pleural surface and located deep in a thickened pleura are usually benign (Fig. 4.25); they typically represent the original surface of the pleura, which has been buried by organization of an overlying effusion. A more florid example of the same process is layered lines of mesothelial cells aligned parallel to the pleural surface. These represent repeated

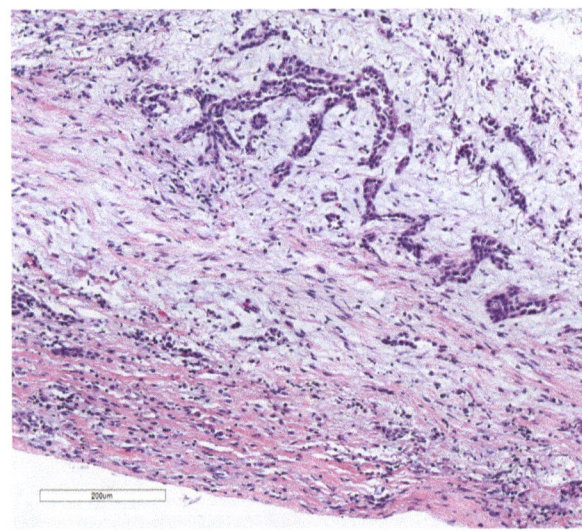

Fig. 4.24 Reactive mesothelial proliferations tend to show a uniformity of growth with entrapment rather than invasive pattern

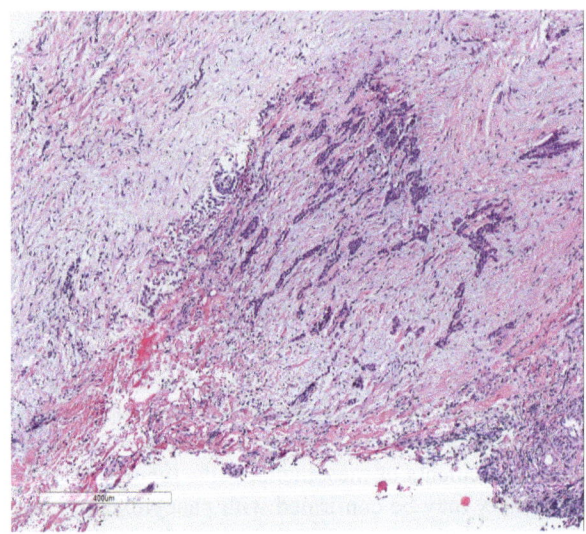

Fig. 4.25 Chronic pleuritis showing lines of mesothelial cells or simple glands arrayed parallel to the pleural surface and located deep in a thickened pleura are usually benign linear layers of entrapment of reactive mesothelial cells

cycles of organization, followed by growth of a new mesothelial layer, followed by further surface organization.

A mesothelial proliferation extending through the whole thickness of a greatly thickened pleura is considered malignant and represents a form of stromal invasion (Fig. 4.26). Another variant is the formation of expansile nodules of stroma, and these can be found within both epithelial and sarcomatous DMM (Fig. 4.21). They may contain relatively few mesothelial cells, but benign processes do not make stromal nodules. Entrapment of mesothelial cells is common and can occur with any type of inflammatory reaction. The inflammation in turn appears to drive

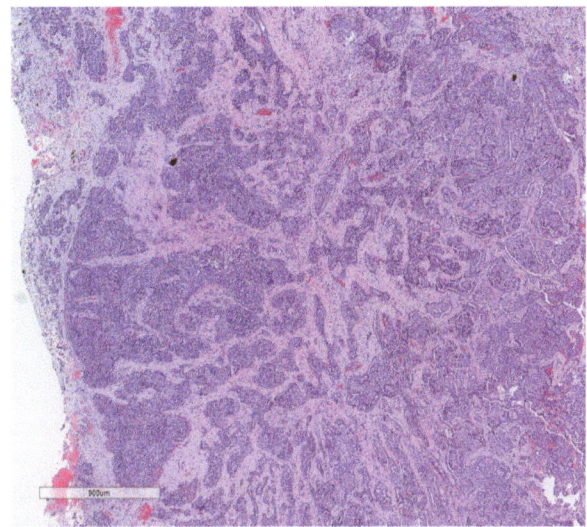

Fig. 4.26 Epithelial mesothelioma showing a complex invasive pattern of solid sheets of tumor cells extending through the whole thickness of a greatly thickened pleura, is really a form of stromal invasion

mesothelial cell proliferations and these can be cytologically quite atypical, a good rule of thumb is to be exceedingly cautious in diagnosing a mesothelioma in the midst of an active inflammatory process especially in small pleural biopsies.

The linear arrays and layered arrays as shown in (Fig. 4.25) are a form of entrapment in which the inflammatory process is usually no longer evident. A helpful hint in circumstances in which there are proliferating mesothelial cells but no inflammation is the distribution of mesothelial cells as mentioned above. Benign processes tend to be sharply circumscribed, with a few glands evident beneath the pleural surface, or with a sharp line beyond which no mesothelial cells are found, whereas mesotheliomas are always invasive with no respect to boundaries.

In summary, separating invasive mesothelial cells of DMM from reactive mesothelial entrapment requires caution. The presence of a significant inflammatory reaction, linear arrays of mesothelial cells, or sharply circumscribed mesothelial proliferations favor entrapped mesothelial cells [39].

Chronic Fibrous Pleuritis Versus Desmoplastic Variant of Sarcomatoid Diffuse Malignant Mesothelioma

Mango et al. [33], studying spindle cell proliferations in the pleura, proposed the key pathologic features important in making the distinction of chronic fibrous pleuritis from desmoplastic DMM, and those features were re-emphasized by others [43]. Identifying one or more of the following features will assist with differentiation: Invasive growth, bland necrosis, frankly sarcomatous areas, and metastatic disease.

Stromal invasion is often more difficult to recognize in spindle cell proliferations of the pleura than in epithelial proliferations. The invasive malignant cells are often

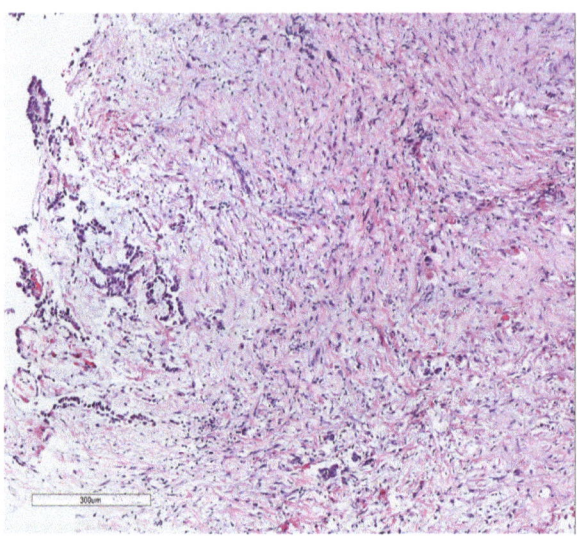

Fig. 4.27 Chronic pleuritis showing zonation phenomenon and entrapped mesothelial cells and the perpendicular capillary arrangements in the fibrous tissue of inflamed pleura

deceptively bland, resembling fibroblasts, and pancytokeratin staining is invaluable in highlighting the presence of cytokeratin-positive malignant cells in regions where they should not normally be present: in the connective tissue, adipose tissue, or skeletal muscle deep to the parietal pleura or invading the visceral pleura and lung tissue as illustrated above. The bland necrosis of paucicellular fibrous tissue by itself may be subtle and one may be reluctant to base a diagnosis of malignancy solely on its presence. Fortunately, most cases that show bland necrosis also show invasive growth. Similarly, the presence of "frankly sarcomatous foci" is a distinctly subjective determination and one would be reluctant to base a diagnosis of malignancy on its presence alone because reactive processes may show marked cytologic atypia, especially at the surface of the process.

Uniformity of growth and the superficial nature of the process with surface atypia and the deep stromal maturation, with perpendicular thin-walled vessels (Figs. 4.27 and 4.28) are typical of chronic fibrous pleuritis in contrast to the disorganized growth pattern and the variable thickness of desmoplastic DMM. A helpful clue in desmoplastic DMM is the presence of expansile nodules of varying sizes with abrupt changes in cellularity between nodules and their surrounding tissue [39].

In summary, the key histopathologic features in separation of chronic fibrous pleuritis from desmoplastic DMM are:

1. Zonation: Chronic fibrous pleuritis exhibits increased cellularity sometime with marked reactive atypia immediately under the pleural effusion and progressively less cellular to paucicellular fibrosis as you move away from the surface (Fig. 4.29). DMM, on the other hand, shows diffuse infiltration of the fibrotic pleura usually by looking bland or sometime by pleomorphic malignant cells with no changes diagnostic of zonation.
2. Invasion: Stromal invasion is the most useful single criterion for separating benign from malignant. In chronic fibrous pleuritis, the fibrosing process is usu-

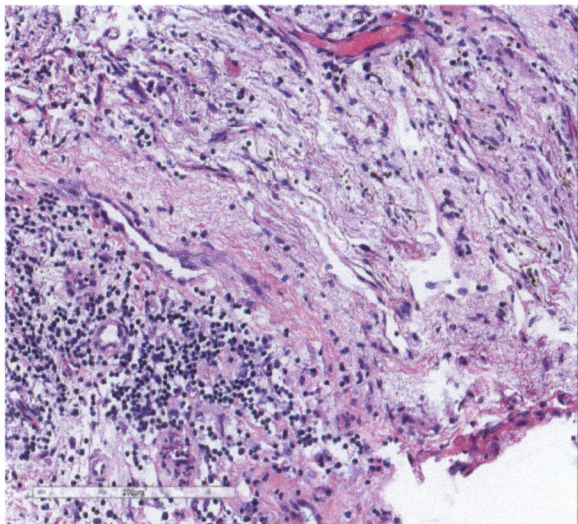

Fig. 4.28 Closer view of the same case showing the perpendicular capillaries arrangements in chronic pleuritis

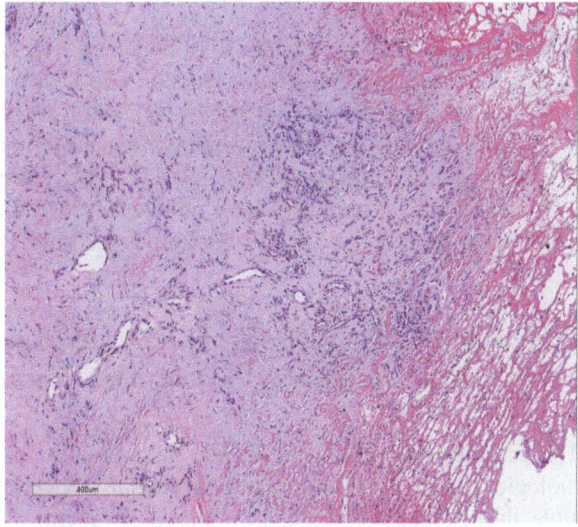

Fig. 4.29 Chronic pleuritis showing the characteristic zonation phenomenon surface fibrin, granulation tissue with capillaries and dense collagen

ally limited to the pleura; whereas in DMM the spindle cells invade the adipose tissue resulting in isolation of individual adipocytes (Fig. 4.20), the spindle cells may also invade muscle and lung parenchyma (Fig. 4.30).
3. Capillaries: The capillaries arising in chronic fibrous pleuritis are typically obvious and usually arranged perpendicular to the surface. With DMM, the capillaries are difficult to see within dense fibrous tissue.
4. Necrosis: Necrosis is usually an indicator of malignancy; however, necrosis may also be seen in benign inflammatory process such as chronic fibrous pleuritis. The necrosis occurring in chronic fibrous pleuritis is rich in inflammatory cells,

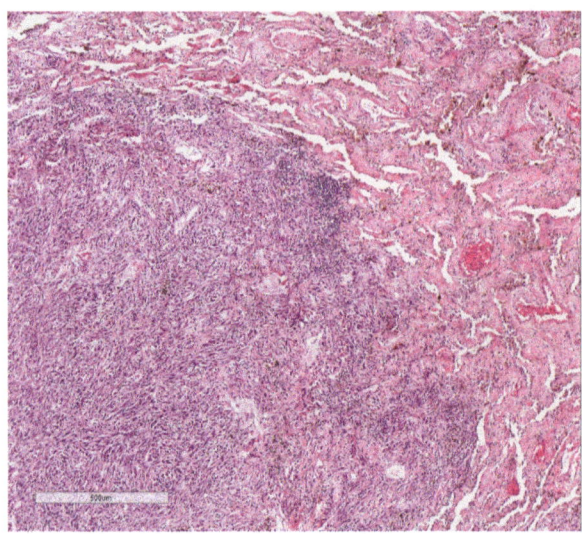

Fig. 4.30 High-power view of the of sarcomatous mesothelioma invading the lung tissue (*right*)

cellular debris, and usually contains few reactive mesothelial cells. The necrosis occurring in DMM is usually sharply demarcated, bland, and infarct-like, with little or no associated cellular reaction and no karyorrhexis or cellular debris (Fig. 4.19), extending into the chest wall adipose tissue or muscle.
5. Nodular stromal expansion: These are expansile nodules of varying sizes with pushing borders and abrupt changes in cellularity between nodules and their surrounding tissue. These expansile nodules if present are diagnostic of DMM and are not a characteristic of chronic fibrous pleuritis.

Sarcomatous Diffuse Malignant Mesothelioma Versus Sarcomatoid Carcinoma or Metastatic Sarcoma

The accurate diagnosis of metastatic sarcoma requires correlation of clinical, radiologic, gross, microscopic, and immunohistochemical information. When possible, the histopathologic and the immunohistochemical studies of the pleural tumor should be compared to those of the primary tumor. Pleural involvement by metastatic sarcoma is typically a late manifestation of the disease, and in most cases a diagnosis of primary sarcoma in the primary location has been established.

Localized Malignant Mesothelioma

Crotty et al. [44] first described a series of six localized malignant mesotheliomas in 1994. Over the years, additional rare cases of localized pleural neoplasms with histopathologic, histochemical, immunohistochemical, and ultrastructural features identical to those of DMM were identified for which the term "localized malignant mesothelioma" is applicable [45–46].

Localized malignant mesotheliomas are extremely rare; grossly the tumor grows out of the visceral or parietal pleural surface as solitary localized pleural masses in a sessile or pedunculated pattern. Most localized malignant mesotheliomas present clinically with nonspecific symptoms. The median age is 62 years. Most reported cases of localized malignant mesotheliomas have been epithelial and biphasic (mixed) type in addition to a rare case of sarcomatous type [45–47]. The differential diagnosis may be problematic, especially if the tumor is histologically composed of predominantly spindle cells. The sarcomatous variant should be differentiated from solitary fibrous tumor (SFT) of the pleura, because SFT are the most common solitary pleural neoplasms, and some have malignant behavior. SFT, histologically, may mimic sarcomatous DMM. Most immunohistochemical studies of SFT have noted that the tumor cells are consistently negative for cytokeratin and positive for CD34 and vimentin. In contrast, sarcomatous DMM is nearly always immunopositive for cytokeratin and vimentin, but not for CD34. It is clinically and prognostically crucial to recognize and separate localized malignant mesotheliomas from diffuse malignant mesotheliomas. DMM always shows gross and/or microscopic evidence of widespread tumor on the pleural surface, which makes its surgical management extremely difficult or impossible. On the other hand, localized malignant mesothelioma in some cases has apparently been cured by surgical excision. Close to 50% of the patients with follow-up in one series [46] were alive, many with follow-up of several years.

References

1. Yates DH, Corrin B, Stidolp PN, Browne K. Malignant mesothelioma in south east England: clinicopathological experience of 272 cases. Thorax. 1997;52:507–12.
2. McCaughey WT, Colby TV, Battifora H, et al. Diagnosis of diffuse malignant mesothelioma: experience of a US/Canadian Mesothelioma Panel. Mod Pathol. 1991;4:342–53.
3. Sporn TA, Roggli VL. Mesothelioma. In: Roggli VL, Oury TD, Sporn TA, editors. Pathology of asbestos-associated diseases. New York: Springer; 2004. pp. 104–67.
4. Boutin C, Rey F, Gouvernet J, Viallat JR, Astoul P, Ledoray V. Thoracoscopy in pleural malignant mesothelioma: a prospective study of 188 consecutive patients. 2. prognosis and staging. Cancer. 1993;72:394–4.
5. Robinson BWS, Lake RA. Advances in malignant mesothelioma. N Engl J Med. 2005;353:1591–603.
6. Elmes PC, Simpson JC. The clinical aspects of mesothelioma. Quar J Med. 1976;45:427–48.
7. Churg A, Roggli VL, Galateau-Salle F, et al. Tumours of the pleura: mesothelial tumours. In: Travis WD, Brambilla E, Harris CC, Muller-Hermelink HK, editors. Pathology and genetics of tumours of the lung, pleura, thymus and heart. Lyon: IARC Press; 2004. World Health Organization Classification of Tumours.
8. Galateau-Salle F, Brambilla E, Cagel PT, et al. Classification and histologic features of epithelioid mesotheliomas. In: Galateau-Salle F, editor. Pathology of malignant mesothelioma. London: Springer-Verlag; 2006.
9. Churg A, Cagle PT, Roggli VL. Tumors of the serosal membranes. Washington, DC: American Registry of Pathology; 2006. Atlas of tumor pathology; 4th series, fascicle 3.

10. Cagle PT. Pleural histology. In Light RW, Lee YCG, editors. Pleural disease: An international textbook. London: Arnold; 2003. pp. 249–255.
11. Galateau-Sallé F, Vignaud JM, Burke L, et al. Well-differentiated papillary mesothelioma of the pleura: a series of 24 cases. Am J Surg Pathol. 2004;28:534–40.
12. Umezu H, Kuwata K, Ebe Y, et al. Microcystic variant of localizd malignant mesothelioma accompanying an adenomatoid tumor-like lesion. Pathol Int. 2002;52:416–22.
13. Arai H, Endo M, Sasai Y, et al. Histochemical demonstration of hyaluronic acid in a case of pleural mesothelioma. Am Rev Respir Dis. 1975;111:699–2.
14. Mayall FG, Gibbs AR. The histology and immunochemistry of small cell mesothelioma. Histopathology. 1992;20:47–51.
15. Cavazza A, Rossi G, Agostini L, et al. Small-cell mesothelioma of the pleura: description of a case. Pathologica. 2002;94:247–52.
16. Dessy E, Falleni M, Braidotti P, et al. Unusual clear-cell variant of epithelioid mesothelioma. Arch Pathol Lab Med. 2001;125:1588–90.
17. Serio G, Scattone A, Pennela A, et al. Malignant deciduoid mesothelioma of the pleura. Histopathology. 2002;40:348–52.
18. Shia J, Erlandson RA, Klimstra DS. Deciduoid mesothelioma: a report of 5 cases and literature review. Ultrastruct Pathol. 2002;26:355–63.
19. Monaghan H, Al-Nafussi A. Deciduoid pleural mesothelioma. Histopathology. 2001;39:104–6.
20. Hammar SP, Bolen JW. Sarcomatoid pleural mesothelioma. Ultrastruct Pathol. 1985;9:337–43.
21. Lucas DR, Pass HI, Madan Sk, et al. Sarcomatoid mesothelioma and its histological mimics: a comparative immunohistochemical study. Histopathology. 2003;42:270–79.
22. Corson JM. Pathology of diffuse malignant pleural mesothelioma. Semin Thorac Cardiovasc Surg. 1997;9:347–55.
23. Yousem SA, Hochholzer, L. Malignant mesotheliomas with osseous and cartilaginous differentiation. Arch Pathol Lab Med. 1987;111:62–66.
24. Okamoto T, Yokota S, Shinkawa K, et al. Pleural malignant mesothelioma with osseous, cartilaginous, and rhabdomyoblastic differentiation. J Jpn Resp Soc. 1998;36:696–1.
25. Suen HC, Sudholt B, Anderson WM, Lakho MH, Daily BB. Malignant mesothelioma with osseous differentiation. Ann Thorac Surg. 2002;73:665.
26. Henderson DW, Attwood HD, Constance TJ, Shilkin KB, Steele RH. Lymphohistocytoid mesothelioma: a rare lymphomatoid variant of predominantly sarcomatoid mesothelioma. Ultrastruct Pathol. 1988;12:367–84.
27. Khalidi HS, Medeiros LJ, Battifora H. Lymphohistiocytoid mesothelioma. An often misdiagnosed variant of sarcomatoid malignant mesothelioma. Am J Clin Pathol. 2000;113:649–54.
28. Cantin R, Al-Jabi M, McCaughey WTE. Desmoplastic diffuse mesothelioma. Am J Surg Pathol. 1982;6:215–22.
29. Colby TV. The diagnosis of desmoplastic malignant mesothelioma. Am J Clin Pathol. 1998;110:135–36.
30. Wilson GE, Hasleton PS, Chatterjee AK. Desmoplastic malignant mesothelioma: a review of 17 cases. J Clin Pathol. 1992;45:295–98.
31. Kannerstein M, Churg J. Desmoplastic diffuse malignant mesothelioma. Prog Surg Pathol. 1980;1:19–27.
32. Churg A, Cagle P, Colby TV, et al. US-Candadian mesothelioma reference panel. The fake fat phenomenon in organizing pleuritis: a source of confusion with desmoplastic malignant mesotheliomas. Am J Surg Pathol. 2011;35(12):1823–29.
33. Mangano WE, Cagle PT, Churg A, Vollmer RT, Roggli VL. The diagnosis of desmoplastic malignant mesothelioma and its distinction from fibrous pleurisy: a histologic and immunohistochemical analysis of 31 cases including p53 immunostaining. Am J Clin Pathol. 1998;110:191–99.
34. Bedrossian CW, Bonsib S, Moran C. Differential diagnosis between mesothelioma and adenocarcinoma: a multimodal approach based on ultrastructure and immunocytochemistry. Semin Diagn Pathol. 1992;9:124–40.
35. Koss M, Travis W, Moran C, Hochholzer L. Pseudomesotheliomatous adenocarcinoma: a reappraisal. Sem Diag Pathol. 1992;9:117–23.

36. Nishimoto Y, Ohno T, Saito K. Pseudomesotheliomatous carcinoma of the lung with histochemical and immunohistochemical study. Acta Pathol Jap. 1983;33:415–23.
37. Dardick I, Jabi M, McCaughey WTE, et al. Diffuse epithelial mesothelioma: a review of the ulstrastructural spectrum. Ultrastruct Pathol. 1987;11:503–33.
38. Wick MR, Loy T, Mills SE, Legier JF, Maniverl JC. Malignant epithelioid pleural mesothelioma versus peripheral pulmonary adenocarcinoma: a histochemical, ultrastructural, and immunohistologic study of 103 cases. Hum Pathol. 1990;21:759–766.
39. Husain AN, Colby TV, Ordóñez NG, Krausz T, Borczuk A, Cagle PT, Chirieac LR, Churg A, Galateau-Salle F, Gibbs AR, Gown AM, Hammar SP, Litzky LA, Roggli VL, Travis WD, Wick MR. Guidelines for patologic diagnosis of maliganant mesothelioma: a consensus statement from the international mesothelioma interest group. Arch Pathol Lab Med. 2009;133:1317–331.
40. Cagle PT, Churg A. Differential diagnosis of benign and malignant mesothelial proliferations on pleural biopsies. Arch Pathol Lab Med. 2005;129(11):1421–427.
41. Churg A, Colby TV, Cagle P, et al. The separation of benign and malignant mesothelial proliferations. Am J Surg Pathol. 2000;24:1183–200.
42. Allen TC. Recognition of histopathologic patterns of diffuse malignant mesothelioma in differential diagnosis of pleural biopsies. Arch Pathol Lab Med. 2005;129:1415–420.
43. Churg A, Galateau-Salle F. The separation of benign and malignant mesothelial proliferations. Arch Pathol Lab Med. 2012;136:1217–1226.
44. Crotty TB, Myers JL, Katzenstein AL, et al.: Localized malignant mesothelioma: a clinicopathologic and flow cytometric study. Am J Surg Pathol. 1994;18:357–63.
45. Okamura H, Kamai T, Mitsuno A, et al. Localized malignant mesothelioma of the pleura. Pathol Int. 2001;51:654–60.
46. Allen TC, Cagle PT, Churg AM, et al. Localized malignant mesothelioma. Am J Surg Pathol. 2005;29:866–73.
47. Gotfried MH, Quan SF, Sobonya RE. Diffuse epithelial pleural mesothelioma presenting as a solitary lung mass. Chest. 1983;84:99–101.

Chapter 5
Immunohistochemistry

Nahal Boroumand

Introduction

Immunohistochemistry has been used to distinguish benign mesothelial proliferation from diffuse malignant mesothelioma (DMM) and to differentiate DMM from other malignancies involving the pleura. DMM has a broad range of cytomorphology and shows a variety of histologic pattern; therefore, distinguishing DMM from other tumors that might metastasize to pleura based on routine histologic preparation is often extremely difficult and without immunostains may be impossible.

Immunohistochemical panels are integral to the diagnosis of DMM, but the exact makeup of the panels used is dependent on the differential diagnosis and on the antibodies available in a given laboratory.

Reactive Mesothelial Cell Hyperplasia Versus Diffuse Malignant Mesothelioma

Distinguishing reactive mesothelial cell hyperplasia from DMM is a major challenge for pathologists. The role of immunohistochemistry for this part is controversial; and histology—especially invasion to the stroma, fat, or lung—is still the gold standard for this distinction. Invasion can be highlighted by immunostains such as pancytokeratin and calretinin. However, in a small biopsy specimen, these features cannot be evaluated.

While there are some immunohistochemical markers that are more likely to be positive in DMM and some that are more likely to be positive in reactive mesothelial cell hyperplasia, currently there is no specific immunostain that can be solely relied upon to make that distinction. Markers that are more likely to be positive

---

N. Boroumand (✉)
Department of Pathology, University of Texas Medical Branch,
301 University Blvd., 2.190JSA, Galveston, TX 77555, USA
e-mail: naboroum@utmb.edu

Table 5.1 Immunohistochemical stains that are used to differentiate benign mesothelial proliferation from malignant mesothelioma

More likely to be positive in malignant mesothelioma
P53
EMA
GLUT-1
IMP3
Claimed to be positive in benign mesothelial proliferation
Desmin

in DMM include P53, epithelial membrane antigen (EMA), glucose transporter 1 (GLUT-1) and insulin-like growth factor II messenger RNA-binding protein 3 (IMP3) [1–5]. Desmin immunopositivity, in contrast, has been claimed by some authors to be more likely to occur with reactive mesothelial cell hyperplasia [1, 2, 6] (Table 5.1). Although review of the literature shows a high specificity of approximately 80–90 % for EMA and P53 with DMM, specificity is nonetheless not adequate for use in differentiating DMM and reactive mesothelial cell hyperplasia. In a recent study by Shi et al., 73 % of DMM were positive with IMP3, while no cases of reactive mesothelial cell hyperplasia stained for it [3]. In distinguishing sarcomatous DMM, especially the desmoplastic subtype, from chronic fibrous pleuritis, cytokeratin plays an important role by exhibiting invasion of chest wall adipose tissue or lung parenchyma [7].

Diffuse Malignant Mesothelioma Versus Other Malignancies Involving the Pleura

The role of immunohistochemistry varies depending on the histologic type of DMM (Epithelioid versus sarcomatous) and the type of the tumor being considered in the differential diagnosis. While some recommendations exist, the number of antibodies necessary for definitive diagnosis or exclusion of DMM is individual to each case.

Epithelioid Diffuse Malignant Mesothelioma

Epithelioid DMM has a broad range of morphologic features and should be distinguished from primary pulmonary adenocarcinoma involving the pleura and metastatic carcinoma arising from other organs.

Because no absolutely sensitive and specific marker for mesothelioma has yet been identified, a panel of immunohistochemical stains composed of mesothelioma markers (i.e., those that are frequently expressed in DMM, but not in carcinomas) and carcinoma markers (those that are frequently expressed in carcinomas, but not DMM) should be used to establish the diagnosis (Table 5.2). The combination of

Table 5.2 Mesothelioma markers and broad-spectrum carcinoma markers

Mesothelioma markers
Calretinin
WT1
D2-40
CK5/6
Thrombomodulin
Mesothelin
Caveolin-1
Carcinoma markers
EP-CAM (MOC-31, BER-EP4)
BG8
CEA (monoclonal)
B72.3
CD15 (Leu-M1)
Claudin-4 (CL-4)

these markers is chosen based on gross and microscopic appearance, radiology, and clinical history. Because none of the markers are 100% specific, the International Mesothelioma Panel recommends that at a minimum 2 mesothelial and 2 carcinoma markers, in addition to a broad-spectrum cytokeratin antibody, be included in any panel [8]. Based on their sensitivity and specificity, calretinin, CK5/6, WT1, and D2-40 are currently considered by many to be the best positive mesothelioma markers; and MOC-31, BER-EP4, carcinoembryonic antigen (CEA), and Lewis (y) antigen blood group 8 to be the best carcinoma markers [1].

In addition to these broad-spectrum carcinoma markers, a number of carcinoma markers are available that their expression is highly restricted to certain type of carcinomas. These markers will be helpful to determine the origin of metastatic carcinomas (Table 5.3).

Thyroid transcription factor-1 (TTF-1) and napsin A are helpful in distinguishing lung adenocarcinoma from DMM. TTF-1 is positive in approximately 75% of lung adenocarcinomas and napsin A in between 58 and 91%; both are negative in mesotheliomas [9–11].

Markers that are helpful in differentiating squamous cell carcinoma from DMM include Ber-EP4, MOC-31, CEA, BG8, and P63 [12]. P63 can also assist in distinguishing squamous cell carcinoma from adenocarcinoma. Of the mesothelioma markers, WT1 is considered by many to be the best marker in this situation, as CK5/6 and calretinin often are positive in squamous cell carcinomas as well as DMM [13].

Other carcinomas that metastasize to the pleura and should be distinguished from DMM include carcinomas of breast, renal, gastrointestinal, ovarian, and fallopian tube origin. Markers frequently expressed by breast carcinomas that assist in differentiating metastatic breast carcinoma from DMM include estrogen receptor (ER), mammaglobin, and gross cystic disease fluid protein-15 (GCDFP-15) [13].

Table 5.3 Carcinoma markers that are highly restricted to some organs

	TTF1	Adenocarcinoma of the lung
	Napsin A	Adenocarcinoma of the lung
		Clear cell and papillary renal cell carcinoma
	PAX8	Renal cell carcinoma
		Serous carcinoma of ovary and peritoneum
	GCDFP-15 Mammaglobin	Breast carcinoma
	CDX2	Adenocarcinoma of GI and pancreatobiliary origin
		Neuroendocrine carcinomas of intestinal origin

However, basal-like breast carcinomas are negative for these markers and frequently express calretinin and CK5/6, making their diagnosis as pleural metastases problematic [14, 15].

PAX8 and PAX2 are useful markers for distinguishing metastatic renal cell carcinoma from DMM because they are expressed in most renal cell carcinomas and generally absent in DMM. Renal cell carcinoma marker (RCC) also might be useful; however, its sensitivity and specificity are significantly lower than those of PAX8 and PAX2 [13].

CDX2 is a sensitive and relatively specific marker for intestinal differentiation. Most of the colonic adenocarcinomas, and adenocarcinomas of small intestine, stomach, and esophagus express CDX2 [16]. In addition, gastrointestinal neuroendocrine carcinomas and carcinomas of the pancreas and biliary tree are typically immunopositive with CDX2; while epithelioid DMM are characteristically CDX2 immunonegative [16].

Sarcomatous Diffuse Malignant Mesothelioma

The role of immunohistochemistry is more limited in sarcomatous DMM than epithelioid DMM. Staining for mesothelial markers is less often positive. D2-40 and calretinin are two mesothelioma markers that are most consistently expressed in sarcomatous DMM in a variable percentage of cases [17, 18]. In a study by Roggli [7], only 31% of sarcomatous DMM were positive with calretinin, and the staining was usually focal with predominantly cytoplasmic and occasionally nuclear reactivity. Expression of CK5/6 or thrombomodulin was also uncommon. Cytokeratin expression is more frequently positive; though. 97% of the cases were immunopositive with CAM 5.2 and CK AE1/AE3.

Pleural sarcomatous DMM must be differentiated from primary pulmonary sarcomatoid carcinoma involving the pleura, and from metastatic sarcomas (Table 5.4). A malignant sarcomatoid tumor that is positive with cytokeratin must include with-

Table 5.4 Immunostains in the differential diagnosis of sarcomatous DMM

Sarcomatous MM	Sarcomatoid carcinoma	Synovial sarcoma	Malignant solitary fibrous tumor
CK+ (usually) Calretinin	CK+ or other ca markers	CK+, focal CD99+, BCL2+ T(X;18)	CK-, CD34+, Bcl2+, CD99+

in its differential diagnosis sarcomatoid carcinoma, sarcomatous DMM, synovial sarcoma, vascular neoplasm such as angiosarcoma and metastatic sarcomatoid renal cell carcinoma. Sarcomatoid DMM can be cytokeratin negative, but it is rare.

The combination of cytokeratin and calretinin immunopositivity is highly characteristic of sarcomatoid DMM; however, it cannot always help to distinguish sarcomatous DMM from sarcomatoid carcinoma and synovial sarcoma. When an epithelial component can not be identified in primary pulmonary sarcomatoid carcinoma distinguishing it from sarcomatous DMM is extremely difficult even with the use of immunohistochemical stains. In this situation, clinical and radiologic findings must be carefully considered in an attempt to establish an accurate diagnosis.

In the setting of a keratin-negative sarcomatous and/or epithelial tumor in the lung, an epithelioid vascular tumor (epithelioid hemangioendothelioma or angiosarcoma), malignant melanoma, and lymphoma must be considered in the differential diagnosis, and a panel of antibodies should be selected to assist in accurate diagnosis. Epithelioid hemangioendothelioma and angiosarcoma are often positive for cytokeratin. CD31 and CD34 will help to distinguish them from DMM. With melanoma, S100 and HMB45 are useful markers; and in lymphoma, CD45, CD3, CD20, and CD30 are useful.

Markers That Are Frequently Expressed in Diffuse Malignant Mesothelioma, but Not Carcinomas

Calretinin

Calretinin is expressed in neurons of central and peripheral nervous system, mesothelial cells, adipocytes, eccrine glands, Leydig and Sertoli cells, ovarian stromal cells, and adrenal cortical cells. It has traditionally been a very popular mesothelioma marker [19]. Calretinin is frequently expressed in all histologic types of DMM, in contrast to other commonly used mesothelioma markers such as CK5/6, WT1, and podoplanin, which are typically expressed in Epithelioid DMM but are often immunonegative in sarcomatous DMM. Calretinin stains both the nuclei and cell cytoplasm (Fig. 5.1). Although neither absolutely sensitive nor specific for the diagnosis of DMM, negative calretinin staining should be regarded as a strong indication for caution in rendering a diagnosis of DMM. Calretinin focally stains a small percentage of adenocarcinomas; however, pulmonary squamous cell carcinomas and small cell carcinoma may be immunopositive with calretinin [20–22].

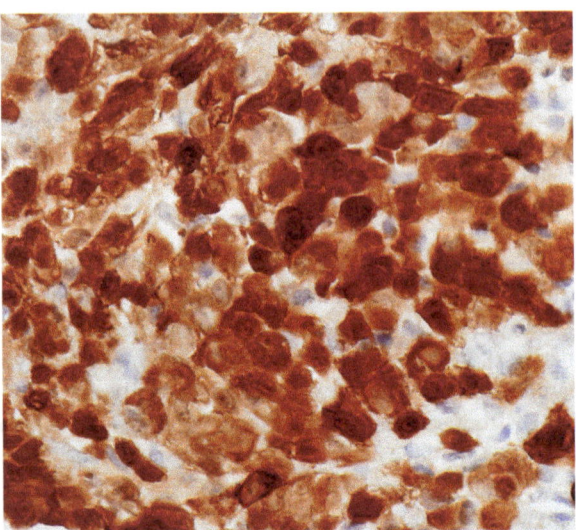

Fig. 5.1 Calretinin stain of epithelial DMM showing nuclear and cytoplasmic immunopositivity

Keratin 5 and 6

Keratin 5/6 Stains positively in almost all Epithelioid DMM; although staining may be focal in some [13]. Keratin 5/6 stains positively in a small percentage of primary pulmonary adenocarcinomas, perhaps due to focal squamous differentiation within the tumors. Keratin 5/6 is not useful in distinguishing DMM from squamous cell carcinoma and breast carcinoma, especially the basal-like breast carcinomas [13, 14].

Podoplanin

Podoplanin is strongly expressed in lymphatic endothelium and a variety of other cells including mesothelial cells [23]. It stains positively in between 86 and 100 % of Epithelioid DMM, and is almost invariably immunonegative in pulmonary adenocarcinomas [24]. The stain has a membranous pattern usually in the apical surface of the cells. Podoplanin is a useful marker in differentiating Epithelioid DMM from lung adenocarcinoma; however, it is not useful in distinguishing Epithelioid DMM from pulmonary squamous cell carcinoma and serous carcinoma. The epithelial component of synovial sarcoma as well as a substantial percentage of angiosarcomas are immunopositive with podoplanin; both of these can be potentially confused with DMM. D-40 is one of the commercially available monoclonal antibodies against podoplanin.

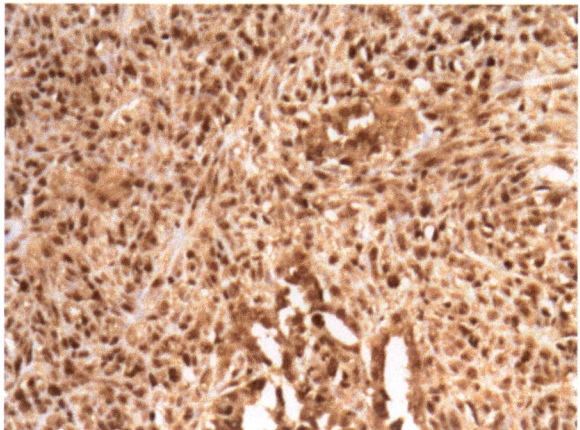

Fig. 5.2 WT1 immunostain of biphasic DMM showing tumor cell staining of both epithelial and sarcomatous components

WT1 Protein

The *WT* gene is located in chromosome 11p13 and plays an important role in the development of the urinary tract, spleen, and mesothelial structures. WT1 is a nuclear stain which is normally expressed in the nuclei of mesothelial cells, sertoli and granulosa cells, decidual cells, CD34 hematopoetic stem cells and glomerular podocytes. Forty three to 100% of Epithelioid DMM are reportedly immunopositive with WT1 [13]. WT1 is a useful marker to distinguish DMM from pulmonary adenocarcinoma and squamous cell carcinoma [13] (Fig. 5.2). WT1 is also useful in distinguishing renal cell carcinoma from Epithelioid DMM; clear cell renal cell carcinoma rarely expresses WT1 [25]. WT1 is not useful in differentiating DMM from serous carcinomas or breast carcinomas.

Thrombomodulin

Thrombomodulin is normally expressed in mesothelial cells, endothelial cells of blood vessels and lymphatics, transitional epithelium, syncytiotrophoblasts and keratinocytes. Seventy five to 80% of DMM exhibit strong immunopositivity with TM, whereas only 8–15% of adenocarcinomas show focal immunopositivity [13]. TM presents a membranous staining pattern (Fig. 5.3). It is not expressed in renal cell carcinomas and therefore it may be helpful in distinguishing these tumors from DMM. Squamous cell carcinomas often, and angiosarcoma and epithelioid hemangioendothelioma on occasion, express TM.

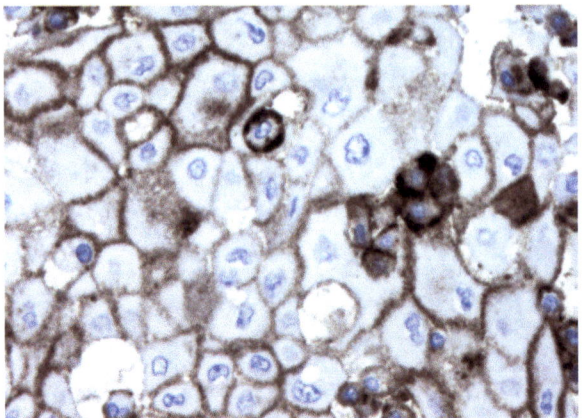

Fig. 5.3 Thrombomodulin stain of epithelial DMM showing membranous staining

Mesothelin

In normal tissue, mesothelin is mainly expressed in mesothelial cells. Some reactivity is also reported in epithelial cells of the trachea, tonsil, fallopian tube, and kidney. Mesothelin is a membranous stain, commonly expressed strongly and diffusely in Epithelioid DMM and adenomatoid tumor. Sarcomatous DMM is usually negative for this marker. Focal cytoplasmic staining with mesothelin has been reported in 40–50% of pulmonary adenocarcinomas and 15–30% of squamous cell carcinomas, so its use in differentiating them from DMM is very limited [26]. Mesothelin is a useful marker for distinguishing renal cell carcinoma and breast carcinoma from DMM. Most pancreatic adenocarcinomas and nonmucinous carcinomas of the ovary, including serous carcinomas, clear cell carcinomas, and transitional cell carcinomas, have been reported to be mesothelin-positive [26]. Mesothelin has high sensitivity and low specificity for Epithelioid DMM; therefore, negative staining for mesothelin strongly militates against the diagnosis of DMM.

Caveolin-1

Caveolin-1 (CAV-1) is one of the most recent markers that has been considered useful in the differential diagnosis of Epithelioid DMM. In a study by Amatya et al., 100% of Epithelioid DMM were positive with CAV-1 whereas only 7.5% of adenocarcinomas expressed immunopositivity [27]. CAV-1 also expressed in 30% of pulmonary squamous cell carcinomas, so is unhelpful in differentiating DMM from squamous cell carcinoma [27].

Type III Collagen

Type III collagen is one of the new and potentially useful markers in differentiating epithelioid DMM from primary pulmonary adenocarcinoma. Further study and validation is required; however, before its routine use can be considered [13].

Broad-Spectrum Positive Carcinoma Markers

Broad-spectrum positive carcinoma markers are immunostains that are positive in wide variety of carcinomas and negative in DMM.

EP-CAM

EP-CAM is an adhesion protein which is normally expressed at the basolateral membrane of the cells in most epithelial tissues including simple cuboidal and columnar, pseudostratified columnar, and transitional epithelium. It is not expressed in adult squamous epithelium, hepatocytes, or myoepithelial or mesothelial cells [28]. EP-CAM is a highly sensitive and specific broad-spectrum epithelial marker; and MOC-31 and BER-EP4 are commercially available monoclonal antibodies against EP-CAM that are commonly used.

MOC-31 is considered to be one of the best positive carcinoma markers, expressed in most adenocarcinomas including lung and breast, serous carcinoma of the ovary and peritoneum, squamous cell carcinoma of the lung, and transitional cell carcinoma [13]. It is only focally positive in a small percentage of epithelioid DMM. MOC-31 is positive in about half of renal cell carcinomas; therefore, it cannot significantly assist in distinguishing between renal cell carcinoma and epithelioid DMM [25].

BER-EP4 is positive in essentially 100 % of pulmonary adenocarcinomas and serous carcinomas of the ovary and peritoneum [9]. It has also been reported to be positive in 87 % of pulmonary squamous cell carcinomas [12] and 42 % of renal cell carcinomas [25]. It may show very focal immunopositivity in small percentage of epithelial DMM. BER-EP4 is helpful in distinguishing epithelioid DMM from pulmonary adenocarcinomas, serous carcinomas, and squamous cell carcinomas; however, it is of little benefit in distinguishing epithelioid DMM from renal cell carcinomas.

CEA

CEA is positive in 50–90 % of pulmonary adenocarcinomas [9] but almost invariably negative in DMM. Because of its high sensitivity and specificity, CEA still is regarded as an extremely useful marker for differentiating these two neoplasms [13]. CEA is also helpful in differentiating pulmonary squamous cell carcinomas and metastatic breast carcinomas from epithelioid DMM. However, it does not assist in distinguishing serous carcinoma and renal cell carcinoma from epithelioid DMM.

Tumor-Associated Protein 72

Tumor-associated protein 72 (TAG-72) was initially identified using the monoclonal antibody B72.3. It is one of the earliest positive carcinoma markers found to be useful in differentiating epithelioid DMM from metastatic carcinoma involving the pleura; about 75–85% of lung adenocarcinomas express positivity with this marker [9]. Approximately, 40% of squamous cell carcinomas exhibit focal positivity for this marker; therefore, it is not useful in differentiating squamous cell carcinoma from DMM [25].

Monoclonal Antibody BG-8

BG-8 is a monoclonal antibody against the blood group Lewis (y). It is reportedly positive in 89–100% of lung adenocarcinomas, 71–100% for breast carcinomas, and 80–83% for squamous cell carcinoma of the lung, while it is negative in most cases of epithelioid DMM [9]. Only 3–9% of epithelioid DMM exhibit focal immunopositivity with BG-8. Most renal cell carcinomas have been reported to be BG-8-negative; therefore, this marker is not useful in distinguishing metastatic renal cell carcinomas from epithelioid DMM [25].

CD15 (Leu-M1)

CD15 is one of the early markers that was used to differentiate epithelioid DMM from metastatic carcinomas. It is essentially always negative in DMM [9]. CD15 is specific but has low sensitivity, immunopositive in only 50–70% of pulmonary adenocarcinomas and 30–60% of serous carcinomas of the ovary and peritoneum [9]. CD15 is positive in most of the clear cell and papillary renal cell carcinomas. It is positive in only 30% of the squamous cell carcinomas, and is therefore unhelpful in differentiating squamous cell carcinoma from DMM [12].

Claudin-4

Claudin-4 (CL-4) is a transmembrane protein located in the tight junctions, that is expressed in most epithelioid cells but is absent in mesothelial cells. It is essentially always negative in DMM, and is positive in more than 90% of the carcinomas. CL-4 is a highly specific and sensitive marker to distinguish epithelioid DMM from metastatic carcinomas [29], and is useful differentiating epithelioid DMM from metastatic renal cell carcinoma [30].

Carcinoma Markers that Are Highly Restricted to Some Organs

There are a few immunostains the positivity of which is highly restricted to only a few organs. Thyroid transcription factor1 (TTF1) is highly restricted to the lung and thyroid gland. It is positive in approximately 75 % of pulmonary adenocarcinomas [9] and is characteristically negative in DMM. TTF1 is a very good marker for differentiating pulmonary adenocarcinoma from DMM. Pulmonary squamous cell carcinomas are characteristically immunonegative with TTF1.

Napsin A is predominantly expressed in the lung and kidney; it is positive in 58–91 % of pulmonary adenocarcinomas [11], in 17–43 % of clear cell carcinomas, and 75–80 % of the papillary carcinomas [11]. Napsin A is characteristically immunonegative in DMM, and therefore can assist in distinguishing pulmonary adenocarcinoma from DMM. Napsin A might also be helpful in differentiating clear cell and papillary renal cell carcinoma from DMM. PAX8 is commonly expressed in epithelioid tumors of the kidney, thyroid, thymus, and some Mullerian neoplasms; however, it is only rarely positive in DMM. As such, PAX8 may help in differentiating renal cell carcinoma and nonmucinous ovarian tumors from DMM [30].

CDX2 is immunopositive in most adenocarcinomas of the colon, small intestine, stomach, and esophagus, and is frequently positive in adenocarcinomas of the pancreas, biliary tree, and neuroendocrine carcinomas of intestinal origin. CDX2 is characteristically immunonegative in epithelioid DMM, and may therefore be a good marker for differentiating adenocarcinomas of gastrointestinal and pancreatobiliary origin from epithelioid DMM [13]. Gross cystic disease fluid protein-15 (GCDFP-15), also known as BRST2, is found in the fluid of fibrocystic breast disease. It is identified in between 23 and 73 % of breast carcinomas [31, 32] and is often expressed in sweat gland and salivary gland carcinomas and in small number of adenocarcinomas of the lung and prostate gland. GCSFP-15 is useful in distinguishing epithelioid DMM from breast carcinomas. Mammaglobin is a breast-associated glycoprotein of unknown function that is expressed in 50–85 % of the breast carcinomas [31, 33]. It is not specific for the breast and can be positive in some cases of endometrial carcinoma, sweat gland carcinoma, and salivary gland tumors. Mammaglobin is not characteristically expressed in DMM, and may be useful in distinguishing DMM from metastatic breast carcinomas involving the pleura.

References

1. Husain AN, Colby T, Ordonez N, Krausz T, Attanoos R, Beasley MB, Borczuk AC, Butnor K, Cagle PT, Chirieac LR, Churg A, Dacic S, Fraire A, Galateau-Salle F, Gibbs A, Gown A, Hammar S, Litzky L, Marchevsky AM, Nicholson AG, Roggli V, Travis WD, Wick M. Guidelines for pathologic diagnosis of malignant mesothelioma: 2012 update of the consensus statement from the international mesothelioma interest group. Arch Pathol Lab Med. 2013;137(5):647–67.
2. Churg A, Galateau-Salle F. The separation of benign and malignant mesothelial proliferations. Arch Pathol Lab Med. 2012;136(10):1217–26.

3. Shi M, Fraire AE, Chu P, Comejo K, Woda BA, Dresser K, Rock KL, Jiang Z. Oncofetal protein IMP3, a new diagnostic biomarker to distinguish malignant mesothelioma from reactive mesothelial proliferation. Am J Surg Pathol. 2011;35(6):878–82.
4. Lee AF, Gown AM, Churg A. IMP3 and GLUT-1 immunohistochemistry for distinguishing benign from malignant mesothelial proliferations. Am J Surg Pathol. 2013;37(3):421–6.
5. Kato Y, Tsuta K, Seki K, Maeshima AM, Watanabe S, Suzuki K, Asamura H, Tsuchiya R, Matsuno Y. Immunohistochemical detection of GLUT-1can discriminate between reactive mesothelium and malignant mesothelioma. Mod Pathol. 2007;20(2):215–20.
6. Attanoos RL, Griffin A, Gibbs AR. The use of immunohistochemistry in distinguishing reactive from neoplastic mesothelium: a novel use for desmin and comparative evaluation with epithelial membrane antigen, p53, platelet-derived growth factor-receptor, P-glycoprotein and Bcl-2. Histopathology. 2003;43(3):231–8.
7. Klebe S, Brownlee NA, Mahar A, Burchette JL, Sporn TA, Vollmer RT, Roggli VL. Sarcomatoid mesothelioma: a clinical-pathologic correlation of 326 cases. Mod Pathol. 2010;23(3):470–9.
8. Husain AN, Colby TV, Ordonez NG, Krausz T, Borczuk A, Cagle PT, Chirieac LR, Churg A, Galateau-Salle F, Gibbs AR, Gown AM, Hammer SP, Litzky LA, Roggli VL, Travis WD, Wick MR. Guidelines for pathologic diagnosis of malignant mesothelioma: a consensus statement from the international mesothelioma interest group. Arch Pathol Lab Med. 2009;133(8):1317–31.
9. Ordonez NG. The immunohistochemical diagnosis of mesothelioma: a comparative study of epithelioid mesothelioma and lung adenocarcinoma. Am J Surg Pathol. 2003;27:1031–51.
10. Ordonez NG. Value of thyroid transcription factor-1, E-cadherin, BG8, WT1, and CD44S immunostaining in distinguishing epithelial pleural mesothelioma from pulmonary and non-pulmonary adenocarcinoma. Am J Surg Pathol. 2000;24:598–6.
11. Ordonez NG. Napsin A expression in lung and kidney neoplasia: a review and update. Adv Anat Pathol. 2012;19:66–73.
12. Ordonez NG. The diagnostic utility of immunohistochemistry in distinguishing between epithelioid mesotheliomas and squamous carcinomas of the lung: a comparative study. Mod Pathol. 2006;19:417–28.
13. Ordonez NG. Application of immunohistochemistry in the diagnosis of epithelioid mesothelioma: a review and update. Hum Pathol. 2013;44(1):1–19.
14. Duhig EE, Kalpakos L, Yang IA, Clarke BE. Mesothelial markers in high-grade breast carcinoma. Histopathology. 2011;59:957–64.
15. Powell G, Roche H, Roche WR. Expression of calretinin by breast carcinoma and the potential for misdiagnosis of mesothelioma. Histopathology. 2011;59:950–6.
16. Kaimaktchiev V, Terracciano L, Tornillo L, et al. The homeobox intestinal differentiation factor CDX2 is selectively expressed in gastrointestinal adenocarcinomas. Mod Pathol. 2004;17:1392–9.
17. Chu AY, Litzky LA, Pasha TL, Acs G, Zhang PJ. Utility of D2-40, a novel mesothelial maker, in the diagnosis of malignant mesothelioma. Mod Pathol. 2005;18(1):105–10.
18. Ordonez NG. D2-40 and podoplanin are highly specific and sensitive immunohistochemical markers of epithelioid malignant mesothelioma. Hum Pathol. 2005;36(4):372–80.
19. Ordonez NG. Value of calretinin immunostainingin diagnostic pathology: a review and update. Appl Immunohistochem Mol Morphol. 2014;22(6):401–15.
20. Mittenen, M, Sarlomo-Rikala M. Expression of calretinin, thrombomodulin, keratin 5, and mesothelinin lung carcinomas of different types: an immunohistochemical analysis of 596 tumors in comparison with epithelioid mesotheliomas of the pleura. Am J Surg Pathol. 2003;27:150–58.
21. Ordonez NG. The diagnostic utility of immunohistochemistry in distinguishing between epithelioid mesotheliomas and squamous carcinomas of the lung: a comparative study. Mod Pathol. 2006;19:417–28.
22. Lugli A, Forster Y, Haas P, Nocito A, Bucher C, Bissig H, Mirlacher M, Storz M, Mihatsch MJ, Sauter G. Calretinin expression in human normal and neoplastic tissues: a tissue microarray analysis on 5233 tissue samples. Human Pathol. 2003;34:994–1000.

23. Ordonez NG. Podoplanin: a novel diagnostic immunohistochemical marker. Adv Anat Pathol. 2006;13:83–8.
24. Chu AY, Litzky LA, Pasha TL, Acs G, Zhang PJ. Utility of D2-40, a novel mesothelial marker, in the diagnosis of malignant mesothelioma. Mod Pathol 2005;18:105–10.
25. Ordonez NG. The diagnostic utility of immunohistochemistry in distinguishing between mesothelioma and renal cell carcinoma: a comparative study. Hum Pathol 2004;35:697–10.
26. Ordonez NG. Application of mesothelin immunostaining in tumor diagnosis. Am J Surg Pathol. 2003;27:1418–28.
27. Amatya VJ, Takeshima Y, Kohono H, Kushitani K, Yamada T, Morimoto C, Inai K. Caveolin-1 is a novel immunohistochemical marker to differentiate epithelioid mesothelioma from lung adenocarcinoma. Histopathology. 2009;55(1):10–19.
28. Winter MJ, Nagtegaal ID, van Krieken JHJM, Litvinov SV. The epithelial cell adhesion molecule (ep-CAM) as a morphoregulatory molecule is a tool in surgical pathology. Am J Pathol. 2003;163:2139–48.
29. Ordonez NG. Value of claudin-4 immunostaining in the diagnosis of mesothelioma. Am J Clin Pathol. 2013;139(5):611–19.
30. Ordonez NG. Value of PAX8, PAX2, napsin A, carbonic anhydrase IX, and claudin-4 immunostaining in distinguishing pleural epithelioid mesothelioma from metastatic renal cell carcinoma. Mod Pathol. 2013;26(8):1132–43.
31. Bhargava R, Beriwal S, Dabbs DJ. Mammaglobin vs GCDFP-15: an immunohistologic validation survey for sensitivity and specificity. Am J Clin Pathol. 2007;127:103–13.
32. Takeda Y, Tsuta K, Shibuki Y, et al. Analysis of expression patterns of breast cancer-specific markers (mammaglobin and gross cystic disease fluid protein 15) in lung and pleural tumors. Arch Pathol Lab Med. 2008;132:239–43.
33. Sasaki E, Tsunoda N, Hatanaka Y, Mori N, Iwata H, Yatabe Y. Breast specific expression of MGB1/mammoglobin: an examination of 480 tumors from various organs and clinicopathological analysis of MGB1-positive breast cancers. Mod Pathol. 2007;20:208–14.

Chapter 6
Molecular Characteristics

Grace Y. Lin

Introduction

The pathogenesis of development of mesothelioma is likely a multifactorial process, with exposure to asbestos considered a major predisposing factor in about 80% of cases. The asbestos fibers are thought to elicit an inflammatory response and reactive oxygen species, which may be involved in genetic mutation, in the mesothelial cells and development of malignant mesothelioma [1]. However, not all people who are exposed to asbestos develop mesothelioma, and other factors such as genetic predisposition have been studied for their possible roles in mesothelioma development. There is a very long latency period of 20–40 years between asbestos exposure and development of mesothelioma, suggesting that multiple mutations must occur for malignancy to develop. Malignant mesothelioma is a rare malignancy, and less is known about the genetic changes than with many other malignancies. Common genetic mutations and other genetic alterations in mesothelioma and the function of the proteins encoded by these genes, as well as possible familial germline mutations that may play a role in mesothelioma development are discussed in this chapter.

Chromosome Abnormalities

Initial karyotyping and comparative genomic hybridization studies have shown mesothelioma to have multiple complex and heterogeneous chromosomal changes. Although up to 44% of cases have been reported to have no chromosomal abnormalities, the majority of cases reportedly have complex karyotypic abnormalities

G. Y. Lin (✉)
Department of Pathology, UC San Diego Health System, 200 W. Arbor Dr. MC8720, San Diego, CA 92103, USA
e-mail: g4lin@ucsd.edu

with hypodiploid and hyperdiploid karyotypes [2–7]. There are regions of some chromosomes which are more likely to contain losses or structural rearrangements [2–7]. (Table 6.1)

One of the most common chromosomal abnormalities described in 29–62% of cases is loss of a region of the short arm of chromosome 9 (9p), most frequently involving bands 9p21–p22 [2, 4, 5, 7, 8] Chromosome 22 or 22q is reported to be lost in 11–57% of cases [2–7]. Abnormalities in the short arm of chromosome 3, in particular, around band 3p21, have been reported in 0–69% of mesothelioma cases [2–7]. These studies have also reported other "nonrandom" chromosomal losses and gains. Subsequent to these studies, various research groups have identified some of the genes present in some of these chromosomal regions and determined the functions of the proteins encoded by these genes.

9p21 Deletion

The most common chromosomal abnormality reported in malignant mesothelioma lies in the short arm of chromosome 9, in particular homozygous deletion of 9p21-p22 [2–8]. This region is lost in many tumor types including melanoma, non-small cell lung carcinomas, gliomas, osteosarcomas, and other tumors [9–13]. The 9p21-p22 region contains the gene for cyclin-dependent kinase inhibitor (CDK) 2A/alternative reading frame gene (*CDKN2A/ARF*), an adjacent related gene *CDKN2B*, and the methylthioadenosine phosphorylase (*MTAP*) gene [9, 14, 15].

Since the initial report, studies have described CDKN2A deletions in 49–80% of malignant mesotheliomas (non-subtyped), 56–77% of epithelioid mesotheliomas, 100% sarcomatoid mesotheliomas, and 84–100% of biphasic mesotheliomas (Table 6.2) [16–22]. In addition mutations in CDKN2A, which lead to loss of function and hypermethylation of 5' CpG islands leading to downregulation of expression of proteins encoded by CDKN2A, have also been described [23]. Because of the frequency of deletion of CDKN2A, identification of CDKN2A deletions by fluorescence in situ hybridization has been suggested as a marker for separation of benign mesothelial proliferations and malignant mesotheliomas, particularly in cytology specimens [19, 24]. CDKN2A may also have prognostic significance; patients that have CDKN2A deletions fare worse than those for whom deletions are absent [23].

The *CDKN2A/ARF* gene encodes two proteins $p16^{INK4a}$ and $p14^{ARF}$.[25–29] $P16^{INK4a}$ is encoded by exons 1α, 2, and 3, whereas $p14^{ARF}$ is encoded by exons 1β, 2, and 3, as well as an alternative reading frame for exon 2 [25–29]. Thus, $p16^{INK4a}$ and $p14^{ARF}$ do not share an amino acid sequence and have distinct binding partners and functional pathways in the cell. However, both $p16^{INK4a}$ and $p14^{ARF}$ are thought to function as tumor suppressors [25–29].

The protein $p16^{INK4a}$ controls the cell cycle via interaction with the cyclin-dependent kinase 4/Cyclin D/pRB pathway. $P16^{INK4a}$ binds to CDK4 and is an inhibitor of CDK4 activity [9, 14, 26]. CDK4 activity leads to activation of cyclins D1, D2, and

6 Molecular Characteristics

Table 6.1 Frequency of nonrandom chromosomal abnormalities of primary mesotheliomas (not including mesothelioma cell lines) by cytogenetics or comparative genomic hybridization (CGH)

Study	Method	Subtype	Normal	3p	9p	Chr. 22	Other
Gibas 1986	Cytogenetics	Epithelioid	1/8 (13%)	4/8 (50%)	3/8 (38%)[a]	Loss chr. 22 2/8 (25%) Translocation 22q 1/8 (13%)	
		Biphasic	0/4 (0%)	3/4 (75%)	1/4 (25%)	Translocation 22q 2/4 (50%)	
		All subtypes combined	1/12 (8%)	7/12 (58%)	4/12 (33%)	5/12 (42%)	Chr 1p, Chr 6, Chr 11, Chr 17
Popescu 1998	Cytogenetics	Epithelioid	0/1		1/1		
		Biphasic	1/1		0/1		
		All subtypes combined	1/2 (50%)		1/2 (50%)		
Hagemeijer 1990	Cytogenetics	Not specified	9/39 (23%)	Loss or translocations 27/39 (69%)	Loss 24/39 (62%)	Loss chr. 22 15/39 (38.4)	Loss 4 q or p Gain Chr. 5, 20
Taguchi 1993	Cytogenetics	Not specified	3/23 (13%)[b]	13/23 (57%)	Loss Chr. 9 2/23 (9%) Loss9p 14/23 (61%)	Loss chr. 22 13/23 (57%)	Chr. 1p and 1q rearrangements 6q, loss of chr. 14, 16, 18
Bjorkqvist 1997	CGH	Epithelioid	2/8 (25%)	0/8 (0%)	4/8 (50%)	Loss 22q 1/8 (13%)	
		Sarcomatoid	1/1 (100%)	0/1 (0%)	0/1 (0%)	0/1 (0%)	
		Biphasic	9/18 (50%)	0/18 (0%)	5/18 (28%)	Loss 22q 2/18 (11%)	

Table 6.1 (continued)

Study	Method	Subtype	Normal	3p	9p	Chr. 22	Other
		All subtypes combined	12/27 (44%)	0/27 (0%)	9/27 (33%)	3/27 (11%)	Loss 4q, 6q, 13, 14q Gain 1q
Krismann 2002	CGH	Epithelioid	3/27 (11%)	Loss chr 3 1/27 (4%) Loss 3p 9/27 (33%)	8/27 (30%)	Loss chr. 22 6/27 (22%) Loss 22q 5/27 (19%)	
		Sarcomatoid	5/28 (18%)	2/28 (7%)	Loss Chr 9 1/28 (4%) Loss 9p21 8/28 (29%)	Loss chr. 22 2/28 (7%) Loss 22q 3/28 (11%)	
		Biphasic	3/22 (14%)	1/22 (5%)	5/22 (23%)	Loss chr. 22 1/22 (5%) Loss 22q 1/22 (5%)	
		All subtypes combined	11/77 (14%)	13/77 (17%)	22/77 (29%)	18/77 (23%)	Loss 1p, 3p, 4q, 4p, 6q, 10p, 17p, 13q, 14q Gains 1q, 7p, 8q, 15q

[a] The study reported that there were 8 cases with chromosome 9 abnormalities, 4 of which were in 9p. Presumably, the remaining 4 were in 9q.
[b] Authors raise the possibility of treatment effect (i.e., no tumor cells left after therapy) or growth of stromal or inflammatory cells rather than tumor cells

Table 6.2 Frequency of *CDK2N2a* homozygous deletion in mesothelioma, polymerase chain reaction (PCR), Southern blotting, fluorescence in situ hybridization (FISH), and/or DNA sequencing observed in studies from various authors who are listed in the first column

	Method	Epithelioid	Biphasic	Sarcomatoid	Biphasic or sarcomatoid	Total
Cheng 1994	PCR and Southern Blotting					5/23 (22%)
Illei 2003	FISH	49/71 (69%)	16/19 (84%)	5/5 (100%)		70/95 (74%)
Takeda 2010	FISH	24/28 (86%)	6/7 (86%)	3/3 (100%)		33/38 (87%)
Bott 2011	Sequencing	20/30 (67%)	6/6 (100%)	3/3 (100%)		29/39 (74%)
Takeda 2012	FISH	23/30 (70%)			12/12 (100%)	35/42 (83%)
Wu 2013	FISH	10/18 (56%)	7/8 (87.5%)	22/22 (100%)		35/42 (83%)

D3 which, in turn, phosphorylate pRB [30, 31] Phosphorylation of pRB releases the transcription factor E2F and, thus, allows transcriptions of numerous genes required for cellular proliferation [30, 31]. Thus, by inhibiting CDK4 activity, p16^{INK4a} slows cell-cycle progression (Fig. 6.1a), and loss of p16^{INK4a} would lead to overly rapid growth for the cells and neoplastic transformation (Fig. 6.1b) [32].

P14^{ARF} likely has multiple functions in the cell, but one major function is regulation of the p53 pathway. Mutations in p53 are uncommon in mesothelioma [20, 33–35]. P14^{ARF} has been shown to interact with and block the activity of mouse double minute 2 (MDM2) and ARF-binding protein 1/Mcl1-ubiquitin ligase E3 (ARF-BP1/Mule; Fig. 6.2a) [36–38]. Both MDM2 and ARF-BP1/MULE are ubiquitin ligases that can ubiquitinate multiple proteins, including p53, and lead to proteasome-mediated degradation of these ubiquitinated proteins [36–38]. P53 is thought to stimulate the expression of another cyclin-dependent kinase inhibitor, CDKN1A/p21 [36–38]. Thus, loss of p14^{ARF} is thought to also allow overly rapid growth of cells and neoplastic transformation (Fig. 6.2b) [36–38].

Subsequently, an adjacent related gene *CDKN2B* which encodes p15^{INK4B}/MTS2 was also identified in this region. About 72% of mesotheliomas show co-deletion of p15^{INK4B}/MTS2 and p16^{INK4a} [39]. P15^{INK4B}/MTS2 is thought to have a similar function as p16^{INK4a} and is an inhibitor of CDK4 and CDK6; thus, p15^{INK4B} is considered a tumor suppressor, which can supplement the activity of p16^{INK4a} in mouse models [40].

MTAP is a gene 100 kilobases telomeric to the *CDKN2A* gene and encodes MTAP. By fluorescence in situ hybridization, *MTAP* deletions were identified in 67% of total pleural mesothelioma cases, 63% of epithelioid mesotheliomas, 79% of biphasic mesotheliomas, and 80% of sarcomatoid mesotheliomas [18]. All of the cases with *MTAP* deletion also showed *CDKN2A* deletion, but about 10% of

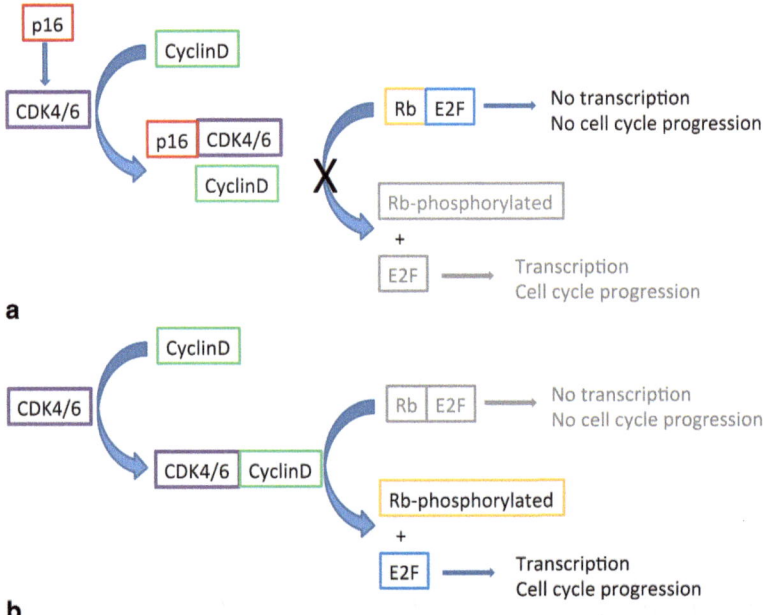

Fig. 6.1 Schematic of p16^{INK4a} function. **a** No deletion of 16^{INK4a}: P16^{INK4a} (*p16*) binds to cyclin-dependent kinase 4 or 6 (*CDK4/6*) and *CyclinD* and prevents phosphorylation of the retinoblastoma protein (*RB*). *RB* remains bound to *E2F* and transcriptional activation does not occur, **b** Homozygous deletion of 16^{INK4a}: Cyclin-dependent kinase 4 or 6 (*CDK4/6*) binds *CyclinD* and phosphorylates the retinoblastoma protein (*RB*). Phosphorylated-RB releases *E2F*. *E2F*-mediated transcriptional activation proceeds and subsequent cell replication can occur

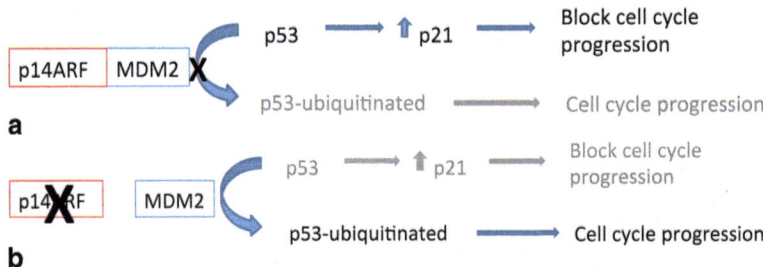

Fig. 6.2 Schematic of p14^{ARF} function. **a** No deletion of *p14^{ARF}*: *P14^{ARF}* (*p14*) binds to mouse double minute 2 (*MDM2*) and prevents *MDM2* from ubiquitinating *p53*. *P53* remains active and can prevent cell-cycle progression or initiate apoptosis, **b** Homozygous deletion of *p14^{ARF}*: *MDM2* from ubiquitinates *p53*. Then, ubiquitinated *p53* is degraded by the proteasome. Subsequently, the cell cycle can progress even in the presence of DNA damage and increase the risk of development additional mutations

cases with CDKN2A deletion did not have *MTAP* deletion [18]. The MTAP protein converts methylthioadenosine to adenine, which is required for AMP synthesis, and methylthioribose 1-phosphate, which is required for methionine synthesis [18].

Chromosome 22

By cytogenetics and comparative genomic hybridization, the most frequent chromosome lost in mesothelioma, occurring in up to 57% of cases, is chromosome 22. In addition, or alternatively, sequences within the long arm of chromosome 22 (22q) may be deleted (Table 6.1) [2, 4–7]. One of the genes present on chromosome 22q12 is *NF2* which is the gene identified in patients with neurofibromatosis type 2. Other genes present on chromosome 22 which also have been reported to be deleted include *SMARCB1, CHEK2,* and *DMC1* [20].

By reverse transcription polymerase chain reaction (RT-PCR) and sequencing, or by fluorescence in situ hybridization, 38–72% of cases of mesothelioma have *NF2* homozygous deletion (both copies of the gene deleted), heterozygous deletion (one copy of the gene deleted), truncations, alternative splice variants leading to deletions of one or more exons, and point mutations or small insertions or deletion leading to missense or nonsense mutations (Table 6.3) [20, 21, 35, 41, 42]. Some reports have indicated that mutations in *NF2* are more common in epithelioid mesotheliomas, whereas other reports have shown increased frequency of *NF2* mutations in biphasic or sarcomatoid mesotheliomas (Table 6.3) [20, 21, 35, 41, 42]. In addition, there is evidence that even in cases with full-length protein expression, the protein is phosphorylated and inactivated [42].

NF2 encodes a tumor suppressor protein Merlin (moesin–ezrin–radixin-like protein) which is also known as Schwannomin or Neurofibromin 2. It was initially identified as the gene involved in patients with neurofibromatosis type 2, which is characterized by development of bilateral vestibular schwannomas, gliomas, meningiomas, schwannomas of other central sites, and juvenile cataract formation [43, 44]. The *NF2* gene encodes at least two main isoforms of Merlin that are found in normal human cells from alternative splicing of the transcripts. Only isoform I is thought to act as a tumor suppressor gene. The function of merlin is complex and the subject of much ongoing research. Merlin is thought to play a role in upregulation and downregulation of multiple signal transduction pathways for cell proliferation. Merlin had been found to interact with at least 34 different proteins [45, 46].

Merlin activity is regulated by phosphorylation. Phosphorylation of serine at amino acid 518 (Ser518) in the C-terminal domain can occur through multiple pathways, including the RAC1 and p21-activated kinase (PAK) pathway as well as by cyclic adenosine monophosphate-dependent protein kinase A (PKA) [46–48]. Phosphorylation of Ser518 leads to unfolding of the N-terminal and C-terminal domains or an "open" conformation. The "open" conformation of the protein cannot interact with many of the proteins to which the "closed" confirmation can bind. Phosphorylation of Ser518 also causes change in localization of the protein from

Table 6.3 Frequency of *NF2* deletion or mutation in mesothelioma by reverse transcriptase polymerase chain reaction (RT-PCR), DNA sequencing, or fluorescence in situ hybridization (FISH) observed in studies from various authors who are listed in the first column

	Method	Epithelioid	Biphasic	Sarcomatoid	Biphasic or sarcomatoid	Total
Bianchi 1995	RT-PCR and sequencing					Mutations 6/15 (40%)
Thurneysen 2009	RT-PCR and sequencing	Mutations and splicing variants leading to truncation 13/26 (50%)	Mutations and splicing variants leading to truncation 4/18 (22%)			Mutations and splicing variants leading to truncation 17/44 (39%)
Bott 2011	CGH, FISH and sequencing					Heterozygous deletion 27/53 (51%)Mutation 4/53 (7.5%) Heterozygous deletion and mutation 7/53 (13%)
Takeda 2012	FISH	Homozygous deletion 10/30 (33%)			Homozygous deletion 6/12 (50%)	Homozygous deletion 16/42 (38%)
Andujar 2013	Sequencing					Mutations including exon deletions and/or point mutations 13/34 (38.2%)

the cell membrane to the cytoplasm [46–48]. The "closed" form of merlin also may function as an inhibitor of the RAC–PAK signaling cascade and prevent PAK-induced cyclin D1 expression [46–48].

Other proteins, such as myosin phosphatase targeting subunit1-protein phosphatase 1δ (MYPT-1-PP1δ), function as phosphatases that can reverse the phosphorylation of Ser518 [49]. In addition, phosphorylation of threonine at amino acid 230 and serine at amino acid 315 in the N-terminal domain, by the PKA Akt may play a role in unfolding of merlin and lead to polyubiquitination and proteasome-mediated degradation [50].

The interaction of merlin with CD44, a cell-adhesion molecule, is thought to be important for inhibiting cell proliferation [51, 52]. The interaction of merlin with the actin cytoskeleton of the cell is thought to be important for cell motility [51, 52]. Thus, loss of merlin or suppression of merlin activity by Ser518 phosphorylation is thought to play a role in cell proliferation, migration, and possibly metastasis.

Merlin may also play a role in the mammalian target of rapamycin (mTOR) pathway, which is thought to regulate protein production, cell growth, and metabolism [53]. Merlin may also play a role in the Hippo cascade, which may also favor cell growth and have anti-apoptotic effects [54]. The Hippo cascade includes SAV1, LATS family members and YAP (see below).

Chromosome 3p21 Mutations: BAP1

By cytogenetics or comparative genomic hybridization, losses of chromosome 3, 3p, or translocations involving 3p were identified in 0–69 % of cases of mesothelioma (Table 6.1) [2, 4–7]. Bott et al. utilized an integrated genomics approach to define copy number alterations followed by sequencing and determined that the gene in 3p21 with the highest rate of non-synonymous mutations was the *BAP1* gene. The *BAP1* gene encodes the BRCA-1-associated protein 1 (BAP1) [55]. Overall, Bott et al. found that 42 % of cases had *BAP1* deletion, mutation, or deletion of one copy and mutation of the other [20]. Sporadic mesotheliomas without germ-line mutations have somatic *BAP1* mutations in 20–23 % of cases (Table 6.4) [20, 56, 57]. Additional reports have found that BAP1 mutations are more common in the epithelioid subtype (13/16) than other subtypes (1/7) of mesotheliomas [58].

Subsequently, Testa et al. reported germ-line mutations in BAP1 in two families with a high incidence of mesothelioma and uveal melanomas [56]. They also found additional somatic mutations in *BAP1* in these family members that led to either loss or mutation of both copies of *BAP1* [56]. Family members with BAP1 mutation were also reported to have breast, renal, pancreatic, and skin cancers [56]. Additional families have also been identified [59]. Testa et al. also found germ-line mutations of *BAP1* in 2/26 patients with sporadic mesotheliomas, and both these patients also had uveal melanomas; no uveal melanoma was identified in the patients without BAP1 germ-line mutation [56].

Table 6.4 Frequency of somatic *BAP1* deletion or mutation in mesothelioma cases without germ-line mutations by comparative genomic hybridization (CGH), fluorescence in situ hybridization (FISH), reverse transcriptase polymerase chain reaction (RT-PCR), and/or DNA sequencing observed in studies from various authors who are listed in the first column

	Method	Epithelioid	Biphasic	Sarcomatoid	Total
Bott 2011	CGH, FISH and sequencing				Mutation alone 6/53 (11%)
					Deletion alone 10/53 (19%)
					Mutation and deletion 6/53 (11%)
Testa 2011	CGH, RT-PCR and sequencing				Mutations 4/18 (22%)
Zauderer 2103	Sequencing				Mutations 24/121 (20%)
Yoshikawa	Sequencing	Homozygous deletion 3/16 (19%)	Heterozygous mutation 1/5	0/2	Homozygous deletion 3/23 (13%)
		Heterozygous deletion and mutation 10/16 (50%)			Heterozygous deletion and mutation 10/23 (44%)
					Heterozygous mutation 1/23 (4%)

Additional studies with more cases are necessary, but there are reports that BAP1 expression may have prognostic significance. One study found that BAP1 mutation status did not correlate with significant differences in survival [57]. However, another study found that the presence of BAP1 protein expression in the nucleus of mesothelioma tumor cells by immunohistochemical staining correlated with a worse prognosis [60]. For uveal melanomas, BAP1 mutation correlates with increased risk of metastasis [61].

The *Bap1* gene encodes BAP1 which was initially discovered through its interaction with the tumor suppressor protein BRCA-1 [55]. Subsequently BAP1 was found to interact with many proteins [20, 62, 63]. BAP1 is a deubiquitinating enzyme which functions as an ubiquitin carboxy-terminal hydrolase within the nucleus [20, 63, 64]. Ubiquitination of proteins within the cell is a tightly controlled process, which targets proteins for proteasome-mediated degradation. Loss of BAP1 function would lead to increased amounts of specific ubiquitinated proteins in the nucleus of cells, and thus increased proteasome-mediated degradation (i.e., decreased amounts) of those specific proteins.

BAP1 interacts with host cell factor 1 (HCF-1) which is a transcriptional cofactor and may play a role in regulation of EF2 and cell-cycle progression [62, 63]. BAP1 forms a complex with the additional sex comb proteins 1 and 2 (ASXL1, ASXL2), and the BAP1–ASXL complex is a member of the polycomb repressive deubiquitinase family of proteins [20, 64]. The polycomb-repressive deubiquitinase family is involved in regulation of histone ubiquitination and may play a role in a role in chromatin modification and gene expression [64].

Hippo Cascade Proteins

As mentioned above, the *NF2* gene product merlin interacts with the Hippo cascade. There are reports of genomic changes for proteins which are downstream of merlin in the Hippo cascade including LATS1 and 2 [20, 65] and YAP1 [66]. LATS1 mutations were identified in 2/53 cases [20]. LATS2 mutations or homozygous deletions were identified in 2/53 (4%) and 3/25 (12%) primary mesothelioma samples [20, 65]. YAP1 which is on chromosome 11q22 has been reported to be amplified in two cases of mesothelioma [64].

The Hippo cascade was initially characterized in *Drosophila* and is thought to be important for regulation of organ size, development and differentiation, and tissue regeneration by restricting cell growth, regulating cell division, and promoting apoptosis [46]. The Hippo cascade includes MTS1/2, Salvador homolog-1 (SAV1), MOB1, LATS 1/2 family of proteins which are ultimately involved in phosphorylation and inactivation of YAP [46]. YAP is transcriptional co-activator, which does not bind to DNA, but instead activates other transcription factors such as p73, Runt-related transcription factor (RUNX), and transcription enhancer activation domain (TEAD) family members [46]. However, *NF2* gene mutation (decreased of merlin activity) in mesothelioma cell lines did not alter YAP1 phosphorylation significantly (suggesting alternative pathways for phosphorylation) [65]. LATS2 mutation did decrease phosphorylation of YAP1 which should lead to increased YAP1 activity [65].

Tumor Suppressor Genes

In addition to the genes that have been identified due to their association with known cytogenetic abnormalities, there has been interest in determining whether common tumor suppressor genes mutated in various other malignancies are involved in the pathogenesis of mesothelioma. The tumor suppressor protein p53, which is involved in cell-cycle arrest and initiation of apoptosis, is mutated in 0–12% of mesothelioma cases [20, 33, 34, 35]. Mutations in other common tumor suppressor genes, including *RB, PTEN* (see below), and *RASSF1,* are also rare [20].

Growth Factor Receptors and Downstream Signal Transduction Cascade

Researchers have also examined the role of growth factor receptors and their signal transduction cascades, which ultimately lead to cell proliferation. Under normal circumstances, the extracellular ligand binds to the growth factor receptor leading to its activation and subsequent activation of the intracellular signal transduction cascade. Some mutations in the growth factor receptor can cause activation of the receptor even in the absence of ligand binding, i.e., constitutive activation. Alternatively, mutation of one of the downstream signal transduction proteins can also lead to constitutive activation of the cascade in absence of ligand binding. For example, mutations in epidermal growth factor receptor (EGFR), a receptor tyrosine kinase, have been reported in a subset of patients with lung adenocarcinoma [67]. In addition, there is interest in EGFR due to the possibility of use of tyrosine kinase inhibitors for therapy [67]. Although EGFR has been reported to be overexpressed in mesothelioma, [68] 0% (0/34 and 0/77) to 16% (6/35) of cases of mesothelioma have been reported to harbor EGFR mutations [35, 69, 70].

EGFR signal transduction can involve several different pathways. One of the pathways involves the mitogen-activated protein (MAP) kinase pathway. The MAP kinase signal transduction cascade involves the RAS and RAF families of proteins. One of the RAS family members Kirsten rat sarcoma (KRAS) has been shown to be mutated in many cancers including colorectal, pancreatic, lung, and breast carcinomas; however, KRAS mutations were rarely identified in 0 (0/34) to 6% (5/77) of mesothelioma cases [35, 69]. The RAF family of proteins includes BRAF. BRAF mutations have been found in many neoplasms including melanoma, papillary thyroid carcinoma, lung adenocarcinoma, and colorectal carcinomas, but BRAF mutations are rare (3/77, 4%) in mesothelioma [69].

Another pathway of signal transduction activated by the receptor tyrosine kinases involves the phosphatidylinositide 3 kinase (PI3K), Akt, and mTOR proteins. PI3K phosphorylates phosphoinositides which then bind to and activate Akt. PI3K has also been implicated in a number of cancers including prostate and breast carcinoma. PI3KCA activating mutations are also rarely (1/77 cases) found in mesothelioma [69]. Phosphatase and tensin homolog (PTEN), which is a tumor suppressor protein, dephosphorylates the phosphoinositides, and thus acts as a brake on this signal transduction cascade. Mutations that lead to loss of activity of PTEN have been described in many neoplasms, including prostate, breast, and endometrial carcinomas, as well as glioblastoma multiforme. PTEN mutations are also rare in mesothelioma [20].

The Search for Germ-line Mutations

Not all people who are exposed to asbestos develop mesothelioma. Several studies have examined whether there are germ-line mutations that increase the risk of development of mesothelioma. An Italian study examined 35 single nucleotide polymorphisms (SNPs) in 15 genes including DNA repair genes, a gene encoding a selenoprotein, and two genes involved in the cellular redox state in people. This study compared sequences from people who developed mesothelioma in a certain high-risk region of Italy and compared those sequences to people from the area who did not develop mesothelioma as well to people from another area of Italy. They identified statistically significant mutations in the DNA repair genes *XRCC1* and *ERCC1* [71]. The protein XRCC1 is thought to be involved in repair of single-strand DNA repair due to ionizing radiation or alkylating agents. The protein ERCC1 is involved in nucleotide excision repair of the damaged DNA. The authors propose that people with germ-line mutations in these DNA repair proteins cannot repair the DNA damage that is induced by the asbestos fibers, and thus are at higher risk of developing other genetic mutations and eventually mesothelioma [71].

In an attempt to identify whether there are any genetic mutations which predispose a person to develop mesothelioma, two case–control studies from Italy and Australia examined genome-wide SNPs for 407 and 428 cases of mesothelioma and 389 and 1269 control patients, respectively. The Italian study examined 370,000 SNPs, and the Australian study examined 2.5 million SNPs. Neither study found statistically significant SNPs nor did they find the same common SNP loci. There were some loci that were more commonly mutated in each of the studies; however, these loci were not replicated by the other study. Additional studies will be necessary to determine if any of these genes play a role in risk of development of mesothelioma [72, 73].

References

1. Liu G, Cheresh P, Kamp DW. Molecular basis of asbestos-induced lung disease. Ann Rev Pathol. 2013;8:161–87.
2. Gibas Z, Li FP, Antman KH, Bernal S, Stahel R, Sandberg AA. Chromosome changes in malignant mesothelioma. Cancer Genet Cytogenet. 1986;20:191–201.
3. Popescu NC, Chahinian AP, DiPaolo JA. Nonrandom chromosome alterations in human malignant mesothelioma. Cancer Res. 1988;48:142–7.
4. Hagemeijer A, Versnel MA, Van Drunen E, et al. Cytogenetic analysis of malignant mesothelioma. Cancer Genet Cytogenet. 1990;47:1–28.
5. Taguchi T, Jhanwar SC, Siegfried JM, Keller SM, Testa JR. Recurrent deletions of specific chromosomal sites in 1p, 3p, 6q, and 9p in human malignant mesothelioma. Cancer Res. 1993;53:4349–55.
6. Bjorkqvist AM, Tammilehto L, Anttila S, Mattson K, Knuutila S. Recurrent DNA copy number changes in 1q, 4q, 6q, 9p, 13q, 14q and 22q detected by comparative genomic hybridization in malignant mesothelioma. Brit J Cancer. 1997;75:523–7.
7. Krismann M, Muller KM, Jaworska M, Johnen G. Molecular cytogenetic differences between histological subtypes of malignant mesotheliomas: DNA cytometry and comparative genomic hybridization of 90 cases. J Pathol. 2002;197:363–71.
8. Lindholm PM, Salmenkivi K, Vauhkonen H, et al. Gene copy number analysis in malignant pleural mesothelioma using oligonucleotide array CGH. Cytogenet Genome Res. 2007;119:46–52.
9. Kamb A, Gruis NA, Weaver-Feldhaus J, et al. A cell cycle regulator potentially involved in genesis of many tumor types. Science. 1994;264:436–40.
10. Fountain JW, Karayiorgou M, Ernstoff MS, et al. Homozygous deletions within human chromosome band 9p21 in melanoma. Proc Natl Acad Sci U S A. 1992;89:10557–61.
11. Brambilla E, Moro D, Gazzeri S, Brambilla C. Alterations of expression of Rb, p16(INK4A) and cyclin D1 in non-small cell lung carcinoma and their clinical significance. J Pathol. 1999;188:351–60.
12. Moulton T, Samara G, Chung WY, et al. MTS1/p16/CDKN2 lesions in primary glioblastoma multiforme. Am J Pathol. 1995;146:613–9.
13. Nielsen GP, Burns KL, Rosenberg AE, Louis DN. CDKN2A gene deletions and loss of p16 expression occur in osteosarcomas that lack RB alterations. Am J Pathol. 1998;153:159–63.
14. Serrano M, Hannon GJ, Beach D. A new regulatory motif in cell-cycle control causing specific inhibition of cyclin D/CDK4. Nature. 1993;366:704–7.
15. Nobori T, Takabayashi K, Tran P, et al. Genomic cloning of methylthioadenosine phosphorylase: a purine metabolic enzyme deficient in multiple different cancers. Proc Natl Acad Sci U S A. 1996;93:6203–8.
16. Cheng JQ, Jhanwar SC, Lu YY, Testa JR. Homozygous deletions within 9p21-p22 identify a small critical region of chromosomal loss in human malignant mesotheliomas. Cancer Res. 1993;53:4761–3.
17. Cheng JQ, Jhanwar SC, Klein WM, et al. p16 alterations and deletion mapping of 9p21-p22 in malignant mesothelioma. Cancer Res. 1994;54:5547–51.
18. Illei PB, Rusch VW, Zakowski MF, Ladanyi M. Homozygous deletion of CDKN2A and codeletion of the methylthioadenosine phosphorylase gene in the majority of pleural mesotheliomas. Clin Cancer Res. 2003;9:2108–13.
19. Takeda M, Kasai T, Enomoto Y, et al. 9p21 deletion in the diagnosis of malignant mesothelioma, using fluorescence in situ hybridization analysis. Pathol Int. 2010;60:395–9.
20. Bott M, Brevet M, Taylor BS, et al. The nuclear deubiquitinase BAP1 is commonly inactivated by somatic mutations and 3p21.1 losses in malignant pleural mesothelioma. Nature Genet. 2011;43:668–72.
21. Takeda M, Kasai T, Enomoto Y, et al. Genomic gains and losses in malignant mesothelioma demonstrated by FISH analysis of paraffin-embedded tissues. J Clin Pathol. 2012;65:77–82.

22. Wu D, Hiroshima K, Matsumoto S, et al. Diagnostic usefulness of p16/CDKN2A FISH in distinguishing between sarcomatoid mesothelioma and fibrous pleuritis. Am J Clin Pathol. 2013;139:39–46.
23. Kobayashi N, Toyooka S, Yanai H, et al. Frequent p16 inactivation by homozygous deletion or methylation is associated with a poor prognosis in Japanese patients with pleural mesothelioma. Lung Cancer. 2008;62:120–5.
24. Illei PB, Ladanyi M, Rusch VW, Zakowski MF. The use of CDKN2A deletion as a diagnostic marker for malignant mesothelioma in body cavity effusions. Cancer. 2003;99:51–6.
25. Quelle DE, Zindy F, Ashmun RA, Sherr CJ. Alternative reading frames of the INK4a tumor suppressor gene encode two unrelated proteins capable of inducing cell cycle arrest. Cell. 1995;83:993–1000.
26. Stone S, Jiang P, Dayananth P, et al. Complex structure and regulation of the P16 (MTS1) locus. Cancer Res. 1995;55:2988–94.
27. Duro D, Bernard O, Della Valle V, Berger R, Larsen CJ. A new type of p16INK4/MTS1 gene transcript expressed in B-cell malignancies. Oncogene. 1995;11:21–9.
28. Mao L, Merlo A, Bedi G, et al. A novel p16INK4A transcript. Cancer Res. 1995;55:2995–7.
29. Ozenne P, Eymin B, Brambilla E, Gazzeri S. The ARF tumor suppressor: structure, functions and status in cancer. Int J Cancer. 2010;127:2239–47.
30. Kato J, Matsushime H, Hiebert SW, Ewen ME, Sherr CJ. Direct binding of cyclin D to the retinoblastoma gene product (pRb) and pRb phosphorylation by the cyclin D-dependent kinase CDK4. Genes Dev. 1993;7:331–42.
31. Kato JY, Sherr CJ. Inhibition of granulocyte differentiation by G1 cyclins D2 and D3 but not D1. Proc Natl Acad Sci U S A. 1993;90:11513–7.
32. Witkiewicz AK, Knudsen KE, Dicker AP, Knudsen ES. The meaning of p16(ink4a) expression in tumors: functional significance, clinical associations and future developments. Cell Cycle. 2011;10:2497–503.
33. Mor O, Yaron P, Huszar M, et al. Absence of p53 mutations in malignant mesotheliomas. Am J Respir Cell Mol Biol. 1997;16:9–13.
34. Kitamura F, Araki S, Tanigawa T, Miura H, Akabane H, Iwasaki R. Assessment of mutations of Ha- and Ki-ras oncogenes and the p53 suppressor gene in seven malignant mesothelioma patients exposed to asbestos–PCR-SSCP and sequencing analyses of paraffin-embedded primary tumors. Ind Health. 1998;36:52–6.
35. Andujar P, Pairon JC, Renier A, et al. Differential mutation profiles and similar intronic TP53 polymorphisms in asbestos-related lung cancer and pleural mesothelioma. Mutagenesis. 2013;28:323–31.
36. Weber JD, Taylor LJ, Roussel MF, Sherr CJ, Bar-Sagi D. Nucleolar Arf sequesters Mdm2 and activates p53. Nat Cell Biol. 1999;1:20–6.
37. Eischen CM, Weber JD, Roussel MF, Sherr CJ, Cleveland JL. Disruption of the ARF-Mdm2-p53 tumor suppressor pathway in Myc-induced lymphomagenesis. Genes Dev. 1999;13:2658–69.
38. Chen D, Kon N, Li M, Zhang W, Qin J, Gu W. ARF-BP1/Mule is a critical mediator of the ARF tumor suppressor. Cell. 2005;121:1071–83.
39. Xio S, Li D, Vijg J, Sugarbaker DJ, Corson JM, Fletcher JA. Codeletion of p15 and p16 in primary malignant mesothelioma. Oncogene. 1995;11:511–5.
40. Krimpenfort P, Ijpenberg A, Song JY, et al. p15Ink4b is a critical tumour suppressor in the absence of p16Ink4a. Nature. 2007;448:943–6.
41. Bianchi AB, Mitsunaga SI, Cheng JQ, et al. High frequency of inactivating mutations in the neurofibromatosis type 2 gene (NF2) in primary malignant mesotheliomas. Proc Natl Acad Sci U S A. 1995;92:10854–8.
42. Thurneysen C, Opitz I, Kurtz S, Weder W, Stahel RA, Felley-Bosco E. Functional inactivation of NF2/merlin in human mesothelioma. Lung Cancer. 2009;64:140–7.
43. Rouleau GA, Merel P, Lutchman M, et al. Alteration in a new gene encoding a putative membrane-organizing protein causes neuro-fibromatosis type 2. Nature. 1993;363:515–21.

44. Trofatter JA, MacCollin MM, Rutter JL, et al. A novel moesin-, ezrin-, radixin-like gene is a candidate for the neurofibromatosis 2 tumor suppressor. Cell. 1993;72:791–800.
45. McClatchey AI, Giovannini M. Membrane organization and tumorigenesis–the NF2 tumor suppressor, Merlin. Genes Dev. 2005;19:2265–77.
46. Sekido Y. Inactivation of Merlin in malignant mesothelioma cells and the Hippo signaling cascade dysregulation. Pathol Int. 2011;61:331–44.
47. Kissil JL, Johnson KC, Eckman MS, Jacks T. Merlin phosphorylation by p21-activated kinase 2 and effects of phosphorylation on merlin localization. J Biol Chem. 2002;277:10394–9.
48. Xiao GH, Beeser A, Chernoff J, Testa JR. p21-activated kinase links Rac/Cdc42 signaling to merlin. J Biol Chem. 2002;277:883–6.
49. Jin H, Sperka T, Herrlich P, Morrison H. Tumorigenic transformation by CPI-17 through inhibition of a merlin phosphatase. Nature. 2006;442:576–9.
50. Tang X, Jang SW, Wang X, et al. Akt phosphorylation regulates the tumour-suppressor merlin through ubiquitination and degradation. Nat Cell Biol. 2007;9:1199–207.
51. Morrison H, Sherman LS, Legg J, et al. The NF2 tumor suppressor gene product, merlin, mediates contact inhibition of growth through interactions with CD44. Genes Dev. 2001;15:968–80.
52. Bai Y, Liu YJ, Wang H, Xu Y, Stamenkovic I, Yu Q. Inhibition of the hyaluronan-CD44 interaction by merlin contributes to the tumor-suppressor activity of merlin. Oncogene. 2007;26:836–50.
53. Lopez-Lago MA, Okada T, Murillo MM, Socci N, Giancotti FG. Loss of the tumor suppressor gene NF2, encoding merlin, constitutively activates integrin-dependent mTORC1 signaling. Mol Cell Biol. 2009;29:4235–49.
54. Hamaratoglu F, Willecke M, Kango-Singh M, et al. The tumour-suppressor genes NF2/Merlin and Expanded act through Hippo signalling to regulate cell proliferation and apoptosis. Nat Cell Biol. 2006;8:27–36.
55. Jensen DE, Proctor M, Marquis ST, et al. BAP1: a novel ubiquitin hydrolase which binds to the BRCA1 RING finger and enhances BRCA1-mediated cell growth suppression. Oncogene. 1998;16:1097–112.
56. Testa JR, Cheung M, Pei J, et al. Germline BAP1 mutations predispose to malignant mesothelioma. Nat Gene. 2011;43:1022–5.
57. Zauderer MG, Bott M, McMillan R, et al. Clinical characteristics of patients with malignant pleural mesothelioma harboring somatic BAP1 mutations. J Thorac Oncol. 2013;8:1430–3.
58. Yoshikawa Y, Sato A, Tsujimura T, et al. Frequent inactivation of the BAP1 gene in epithelioid-type malignant mesothelioma. Cancer Sci. 2012;103:868–74.
59. Cheung M, Talarchek J, Schindeler K, et al. Further evidence for germline BAP1 mutations predisposing to melanoma and malignant mesothelioma. Cancer Genet. 2013;206:206–10.
60. Arzt L, Quehenberger F, Halbwedl I, Mairinger T, Popper HH. BAP1 Protein is a Progression Factor in Malignant Pleural Mesothelioma. Pathol Oncol Res. 2014;20(1):145–51.
61. Harbour JW, Onken MD, Roberson ED, et al. Frequent mutation of BAP1 in metastasizing uveal melanomas. Science. 2010;330:1410–3.
62. Machida YJ, Machida Y, Vashisht AA, Wohlschlegel JA, Dutta A. The deubiquitinating enzyme BAP1 regulates cell growth via interaction with HCF-1. J Biol Chem. 2009;284:34179–88.
63. Misaghi S, Ottosen S, Izrael-Tomasevic A, et al. Association of C-terminal ubiquitin hydrolase BRCA1-associated protein 1 with cell cycle regulator host cell factor 1. Mol Cell Biol. 2009;29:2181–92.
64. Scheuermann JC, de Ayala Alonso AG, Oktaba K, et al. Histone H2A deubiquitinase activity of the Polycomb repressive complex PR-DUB. Nature. 2010;465:243–7.
65. Murakami H, Mizuno T, Taniguchi T, et al. LATS2 is a tumor suppressor gene of malignant mesothelioma. Cancer Res. 2011;71:873–83.

66. Yokoyama T, Osada H, Murakami H, et al. YAP1 is involved in mesothelioma development and negatively regulated by Merlin through phosphorylation. Carcinogenesis. 2008;29:2139–46.
67. Paez JG, Janne PA, Lee JC, et al. EGFR mutations in lung cancer: correlation with clinical response to gefitinib therapy. Science. 2004;304:1497–500.
68. Destro A, Ceresoli GL, Falleni M, et al. EGFR overexpression in malignant pleural mesothelioma. An immunohistochemical and molecular study with clinico-pathological correlations. Lung Cancer. 2006;51:207–15.
69. Mezzapelle R, Miglio U, Rena O, et al. Mutation analysis of the EGFR gene and downstream signalling pathway in histologic samples of malignant pleural mesothelioma. Brit J Cancer. 2013;108:1743–9.
70. Enomoto Y, Kasai T, Takeda M, et al. Epidermal growth factor receptor mutations in malignant pleural and peritoneal mesothelioma. J Clin Pathol. 2012;65:522–7.
71. Betti M, Ferrante D, Padoan M, et al. XRCC1 and ERCC1 variants modify malignant mesothelioma risk: a case-control study. Mutat Res. 2011;708:11–20.
72. Cadby G, Mukherjee S, Musk AW, et al. A genome-wide association study for malignant mesothelioma risk. Lung Cancer. 2013;82:1–8.
73. Matullo G, Guarrera S, Betti M, et al. Genetic variants associated with increased risk of malignant pleural mesothelioma: a genome-wide association study. PloS one. 2013;8:e61253.

Chapter 7
Therapy

Eric Bernicker, Puja Gaur, Snehal Desai, Bin S. Teh
and Shanda H. Blackmon

Introduction

Malignant mesotheliomas are aggressive tumors that arise from serosal cells of the pleural, peritoneal, and occasionally the pericardial surfaces. While the US incidence is declining since the decreased use of asbestos in building [1], the worldwide incidence is increasing and expected to peak in the next 10–20 years [2]. There is a long latency period from the exposure to asbestos, the primary etiological factor of the disease, to the development of clinical symptoms [3–8]. In this chapter, we review the various treatment options of surgery, radiation therapy, and chemotherapy, and discuss the evolving use of a multidisciplinary approach to therapy. Lastly, we discuss some possible novel therapeutic approaches that are being developed and studied.

Role of Surgery

Given that there are limited chemotherapy and/or biologic agents that are effective for malignant pleural mesothelioma (MPM), thoracic surgery often plays a major role in terms of cytoreduction as long as the tumor burden is confined to one pleural space [9]. If the tumor is too advanced and/or invades the heart, mediastinal

---

E. Bernicker (✉)
Cancer Center, Houston Methodist Hospital, 6445 Main Street Floor 21,
Houston, TX 77030, USA
e-mail: Bernicker@houstonmethodist.org

P. Gaur · S. H. Blackmon
Department Thoracic Surgery, Houston Methodist Hospital, Houston, TX, USA

S. Desai · B. S. Teh
Department of Radiation Oncology, Houston Methodist Hospital, Houston, TX, USA

© Springer Science+Business Media New York 2015
T. C. Allen (ed.), *Diffuse Malignant Mesothelioma*, DOI 10.1007/978-1-4939-2374-8_7

vascular structures, or spine, it is considered nonresectable, and patients are usually referred for definitive chemotherapy with or without radiation for local symptoms. The two surgical options that are typically offered to patients are either a pleurectomy/decortication (P/D) or a radical approach of extrapleural pneumonectomy (EPP). P/D is usually offered to patients with early-stage disease where the tumor is confined to the pleura only and the tumor is stripped off the lung by removing the visceral and parietal pleura, thus sparing the lung parenchyma [10]. The other radical approach is an EPP where the entire lung is removed with the parietal pleura en bloc due to excessive tumor burden involving the lung parenchyma, lobar fissures, and/or double-digit nodal station (levels 10–14) involvement.

The typical workup of a patient who is being evaluated for surgery is for the most part universal among institutions. These surgeries are usually performed in a tertiary-care hospital in an academic setting where the intensive care unit (ICU) and thoracic nursing staff are appropriately trained on managing the patients postoperatively. When the patient is first assessed by a thoracic surgeon in clinic, he/she evaluates the patient's tumor burden by reviewing available imaging that typically is composed of a chest computerized tomography (CT) and positron emission tomography (PET) scan. If chest wall or vertebral inversion is suspected, the surgeon may order a chest magnetic resonance imaging (MRI) to evaluate for bony and soft-tissue invasion. If the tumor is too diffuse or the patient has any of the poor prognostic factors as shown in the literature—such as male gender, older age, mixed or sarcomatoid histology, and N2 disease—the risks and benefits of surgical options are weighed against each other [11–13]. The patient must be an appropriate surgical candidate and his/her comorbidities are considered prior to committing the patient to any surgical procedure. Patients with MPM often have exposure to smoke and dust in addition to asbestos that can give them resultant chronic obstructive pulmonary disease (COPD) and emphysema, which can compromise their recovery. Additionally, a fraction of the patients also present with cardiac disease secondary to underlying pulmonary hypertension that may have gone unnoticed for years prior to presentation. All these comorbidities are thoroughly evaluated prior to performing either of these surgeries and patients are medically optimized before surgical resection is performed.

Once the patient's history has been thoroughly reviewed, and the patient is deemed appropriate for surgery, the patient is set staged by undergoing either an endoscopic bronchial ultrasound (EBUS) or a cervical mediastinoscopy (C-med) to rule out mediastinal lymph node disease. Over the years, several staging systems for MPM have been proposed; however, the tumor—lymph node—metastasis (TNM) staging is perhaps the most universally accepted staging system (Table 7.1) [14]. If the patient is found to have mediastinal (level N2 or N3) disease, they are treated with neoadjuvant chemotherapy that typically includes 4–6 cycles of cisplatin and pemetrexed (discussed further below), followed by restaging scans and EBUS or C-med. If the tumor gets downstaged, the patient may be offered surgical resection with or without resection and reconstruction of pericardium and/or diaphragm depending on the extent of tumor involvement.

Table 7.1 TNM staging for malignant pleural mesothelioma (MPM)

T1	Tumor limited to ipsilateral parietal pleura
T1a	No involvement of visceral pleura
T1b	Some scattered foci involving visceral pleura
T2	Tumor involving entire ipsilateral pleura, both visceral and parietal
	Plus, invasion of diaphragmatic muscle
	Or, confluent involvement of visceral pleura, including the fissures
	Or, invasion from visceral pleura into pulmonary parenchyma
T3	Tumor locally advanced but potentially resectable
T4	Tumor locally advanced but technically unresectable
NX	Regional nodes cannot be assessed
N0	No lymph node metastasis
N1	Metastasis to ipsilateral bronchopulmonary or hilar lymph nodes
N2	Metastasis to subcarinal or ipsilateral mediastinal nodes
N3	Metastasis to contralateral mediastinal or internal mammary nods, or to any supraclavicular node
MX	Distant metastasis cannot be assessed
M0	No distant metastasis
M1	Distant metastasis present
Stage	*Description*
Stage I	
Ia	T1aN0M0
Ib	T1bN0M0
Stage II	T2N0M0
Stage III	Any T3M0
	Any N1M0
	Any N2M0
Stage IV	Any T4
	Any N3
	Any M1

EPP is a complex operation where the lung, pleura, pericardium, and diaphragm are resected en bloc [15]. It is performed via a single-extended posterolateral thoracotomy that is then followed by careful extrapleural dissection that is carried over up to the apex of the chest and peeled off the subclavian vessels around the hilum and down to the central tendon. On the left, the aorta is evaluated for possible invasion and care is taken while removing tumor from the aortopulmonary window by ensuring that the recurrent laryngeal nerve is preserved. On the right, care is taken to avoid avulsion of the azygos and injuring the thoracic duct, which can also be ligated to avoid getting a postoperative chyle leak. The phrenic nerve is typically visualized and preserved unless the tumor encases the nerve or the diaphragm is involved which would require its resection anyway, and hence preservation of the phrenic nerve is not necessary. Occasionally, the superior vena cava can have tumor involvement that can be resected and reconstructed with or without the assistance of a cardiovascular surgeon. Pulmonary vein and arterial dissection around the hilum is carried out carefully and if the hilum seems to be too difficult to dissect, an intrapericardial pneumonectomy may be warranted. The bronchus is divided and either sewn or stapled; the margins are checked intraoperatively. Once deemed clear of tumor, the bronchial stump is typically covered with either omentum, intercostal muscle harvested during the thoracotomy, or pleura.

A P/D, on the other hand, starts off with an extrapleural dissection but eventually requires entering the pleural space and carefully removing the parietal and visceral pleura [15]. If the pericardium or diaphragm is noted to be involved on either side, they are resected to achieve negative margins. In order to prevent cardiac herniation, a fenestrated prosthetic patch (Goretex, W.L. Gore and Associates, Flagstaff, AZ) is placed and anchored circumferentially to prevent pericardial effusion and tamponade. The diaphragm is also reconstructed with two pieces of prosthetic mesh that are overlapped to create a dynamic seam and prevent herniation of abdominal contents into the chest. The patch is then secured to the chest wall, central tendon, and pericardium circumferentially using 0-Ethibond sutures. Usually, if the institution offers intraoperative chemotherapy, the pericardial and diaphragmatic reconstruction is saved for after completion of intrapleural chemotherapy treatment (see below).

Because local recurrence limits patient survival in this disease, recent studies have studied and demonstrated that intrapleural heated chemotherapy administered at the time of surgery, can extend interval to recurrence (27.1 vs. 12.8 months), and patient survival (35.3 vs. 22.8 months) [16, 17]. This heated intraoperative chemotherapy (HIOC) protocol entails administering cisplatin as a 1-h lavage of the chest and/or abdomen, in case of diaphragmatic resection, at 42° after completion of EPP or P/D, when minimal tumor burden is present. The toxic effects of the drug are balanced with the administration of intravenous (IV) sodium thiosulfate and amifostine. Argon beam is used to ablate the chest wall, mediastinal wall, and diaphragm after the HIOC run to attain microscopic cytoreduction of any disease left behind.

There are multiple potential complications that are associated with either surgical approach. The most common ones that we encounter are postoperative dysrhythmias, myocardial infarction, prolonged intubation secondary to air leak, aspiration, or acute respiratory distress syndrome, deep venous thrombosis and pulmonary embolism requiring either anticoagulation or inferior vena cava (IVC) filter placement, pulmonary hypertension, vocal cord paralysis, stroke, empyema, bronchopleural fistula, and patch dehiscence requiring a return trip to the operating room. Postoperative renal failure is another potential risk from the HIOC despite the pharmacologic protection.

The goal of surgery in the multimodality treatment of MPM is to dramatically reduce tumor burden such that tumor ablation with the argon beam and HIOC can potentially eradicate microscopic disease, and thereby decrease the incidence of tumor recurrence. Although surgery is offered to patients with MPM, clinicians should caution offering these surgeries to patients with poor prognostic features, advanced disease, and mediastinal node involvement, as these patients demonstrate poor long-term survival.

Radiation Therapy

Radiation therapy uses high-energy X-rays to kill cancer cells. More than 50% of cancer patients receive radiation therapy as part as their overall treatment plan. Patients usually receive external-beam radiation therapy in daily treatment sessions (5 days a week) over the course of several weeks. The number of treatment sessions depends on the treatment intent, cancer type, stage, and patient's performance status (PS).

Radiation is used in the treatment of MPM mainly for local control. It can be used for radical treatment, part of multimodality treatment after P/D or EPP as well as palliation. However, treatment with radiation therapy in MPM is hampered by the challenge to deliver tumoricidal doses while minimizing toxicity. This is owing to the large volume to be irradiated including the entire hemithorax with many adjacent critical radiosensitive structures (heart, lung, spinal cord).

The target volume of adjuvant radiation therapy after pleurectomy or EPP includes the entire visceral and parietal pleura of the side involved. This includes not only the outer lung surface but also along the fissures in cases of pleurectomy alone. Because the lung remains in place after pleurectomy, radiation doses must be lower than when EPP is performed [18]. Initial treatment of the hemithorax with radiation delivered using a photon/electron combination was developed at Memorial Sloan Kettering Cancer Center (MSKCC) in the 1980s [19]. In this technique, a radiation block is used to shield the central portion of the lung, heart, spinal cord, and liver, which limits the total dose to the pleural surfaces.

Even after oncologic surgical procedures, there is a high rate of local recurrences. There have been numerous reports of the use of adjuvant radiation therapy after pleurectomy using the photon/electron match technique in which areas of the target receive less than the prescribed dose. The largest study was published by Gupta where the mean radiation dose was 42.5–45 Gy [20]. Unfortunately, the median survival was only 13.5 months with 28% of patients developing grade 3–4 toxicity after radiation therapy and a palliative surgical procedure. Radiation therapy after EPP is also complex, however, since the entire ipsilateral lung is removed; this does provide a certain advantage by decreasing the potential toxicity from pneumonitis. Using conventional radiation techniques with the photon/electron match technique, the MSKCC group showed promising results [21]. In a phase II trial of induction chemotherapy, EPP, and postoperative radiation therapy, median survival of 33.5 months was achieved, and there was no patient with grade 3 or higher toxicity [22].

Despite improvement in local control with adjuvant conventional radiation therapy, local control and toxicity rates were not ideal. The field of radiation therapy has advanced significantly over two decades with new technology and planning systems allowing for complicated treatment planning and delivery. Intensity-modulated radiation therapy (IMRT) improves the efficacy of higher radiation doses to the entire target volume while minimizing radiation dose to critical surrounding structures by creating a highly conformal radiation plan (Fig. 7.1). Recent advances with image-guided radiation therapy (IGRT), have improved the accuracy of radiation delivery, and thus reduced the treatment margin leading to further decrease in the

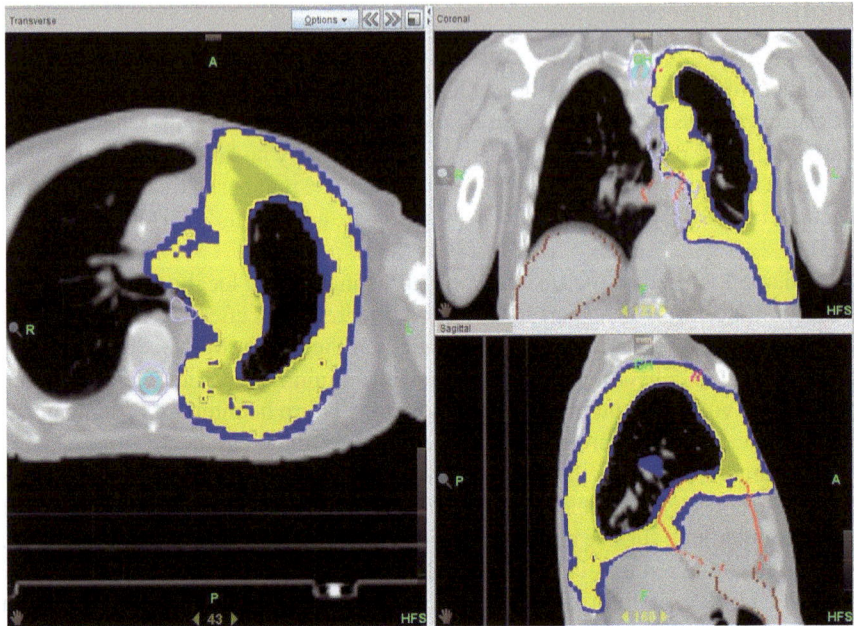

Fig. 7.1 An example of IMRT treatment planning

volume of normal tissues receiving high-dose radiation. The reduction of radiation dose to normal structures allows for decreased toxicity involving all critical organs, especially the lungs.

Initial multimodality treatment using IMRT showed troubling results with increased pulmonary toxicity of the single lung. MD Anderson Cancer Center (MDACC) used IMRT by dose-escalating patients after EPP to 50 Gy with a boost to 60 Gy to positive margins. In an updated MDACC publication by Rice, the local recurrence rate for 63 patients treated with IMRT after EPP was only 13%; however, early mortality was significant with 23 deaths within 6 months [23]. Another early study using IMRT supported lower recurrence rate of 14% vs. 42% for patients treated with conventional radiation therapy [24]. The Dana–Farber group also reported 46% fatal pulmonary toxicity in patients treated with IMRT after EPP [25]. Due to the unexpectedly high pulmonary toxicity due to radiation dose to the contralateral intact lung, a toxicity analysis study found that the volume of lung receiving 20 Gy (V20) and the mean lung dose (MLD) must be kept as low as possible with recommendations of MLD<8.5 Gy and V20<7% [26, 27].

Recent studies from experienced centers have shown safe adjuvant IMRT delivery even in the presence of the intact lung [28–30]. A prospective Italian study involving 20 patients after radical pleurectomy, receiving high-dose radiation to 50 Gy with boost to 60 Gy, showed 3-year local control of 60% without fatal toxicity. Only five patients had grade 2–3 pneumonitis [29]. Gomez also published results from an updated series from MDACC of 86 patients treated with IMRT after

EPP. At 2 years, the rate of overall survival (OS) was 32% with local control of 55%. However, the grade 3 or higher pulmonary toxicity was 11.6% [30]. Even in expert centers with improved techniques, expected rates of grade 3 or worse radiation pneumonitis are 12–20%, and the rates of fatal pneumonitis are approximately 3–8% [31].

Patients with advanced or recurrent disease suffer from symptoms of pain, dyspnea, and esophageal symptoms. Radiation therapy can be used to palliate both the local and distant symptoms as it is used in other cancers. Most of the literature, both retrospective and prospective, has reported a 50–70% response rate of using palliative radiotherapy in MPM. Various palliative dose regimens have been used showing a dose response to pain control with individual doses greater than 4 Gy. Unfortunately, the pain control is short lived with median time to pain recurrence of 2 months [32].

Chemotherapy for MPM

A number of cytotoxic agents have modest single-agent activity against mesothelioma, including the platinum agents, antifolates such as pemetrexed and raltitrexed, anthracyclines, and the spindle toxin vinorelbine. Most agents that have been tested have relatively low response rates, generally between 10–20%, when utilized as a single-agent except for cisplatin and the antifolates, and for that reason, combination cytotoxic therapy has been the primary chemotherapeutic strategy tested over the recent past [33].

Byrne and colleagues reported on a combination of cisplatin and gemcitabine [34]. The cisplatin was given at a dose of 100 mg/m^2 on day 1, and the gemcitabine was administered 1000 mg/m^2 IV on days 1, 8, and 15. Tolerance of the regimen was good, with the main toxicities being hematologic and gastrointestinal. Ten of 21 patients had objective responses (47.6%) and an additional 9 patients had stable disease. While the trial was not designed to assess for quality of life, all responding patients reported an improvement in disease-related symptoms. The 1-year estimated survival was 41%. Based on these promising results, a multicenter confirmatory trial was performed [35]. The partial response (PR) rate was 33%, and 60% of patients had stable disease; the median survival from initiation of chemotherapy was over 11 months. All responding patients had significant improvements in quality of life.

Pemetrexed is a multitargeted antifolate that has significant activity against mesothelioma [36]. In an early phase I study, where the study drug was partnered with cisplatin, there were four out of ten PRs in patients with MPM [37]. This eventually led to a phase 3 trial, comparing the combination of pemetrexed plus cisplatin to cisplatin alone, in patients with advanced MPM [38]. There were three early treatment-related deaths on the pemetrexed arm, and the protocol was modified so that B12 and folic acid supplementation were required after data suggested a significant decrease in toxicity. Two-thirds of the patients had epithelial histology and 78% had stage III or IV disease. The median survival was significantly improved in the combination arm: 12.1 vs. 9.3 months, and the vitamin supplementation improved tolerance without adversely affecting efficacy. Based on this, pemetrexed and cisplatin became the standard of care for frontline therapy for patients with advanced disease.

The combination of cisplatin with a different antifolate agent was also demonstrated to be active with raltitrexed—a quinazoline folate analog that acts as a pure and specific thrymidine synthetase inhibitor. In a randomized trial pairing raltitrexed with cisplatin vs. cisplatin monotherapy, there was a significant improvement in survival, 11.4 months to 8.8, similar in magnitude to the benefit seen with pemetrexed [39]. Stable disease was similar in both arms (54 and 53 %) and toxicity was manageable with no decreases in the health-related quality of life (HRQOL).

Because of the toxicities associated with cisplatin, such as nausea and vomiting, nephrotoxicity, and neuropathy, alternative agents to pair with pemetrexed were sought. Janne et al. reported on a combination of pemetrexed with gemcitabine using two different dosing schemes [40]. The results were disappointing, with the response rates less than those achieved with pemetrexed and cisplatin, and the median survivals being less as well than those achieved with single-agent pemetrexed. While the median age of patients were higher than on the Vogelzang trial, and more had stage IV disease, it still suggested that the gold standard was a platinum doublet with an antifolate.

Because of its more favorable toxicity profile, carboplatin has been studied in combination with pemetrexed. Ceresoli et al. reported on the results of a phase II study, giving pemetrexed at a standard dose of 500 mg/m^2 along with carboplatin dosed to an area under the curve of 5 [41]. All patients received vitamin supplementation with B12 and folic acid. The response rate was 18.6 % and an additional 47 % had disease stabilization. The median survival compared favorably with that achieved with pemetrexed and cisplatin—12.7 months. Not surprisingly, the non-hematological toxicity was negligible, suggesting that this combination might be useful in older patients with MPM or those with significant comorbid conditions.

The development of vascular endothelial growth factor (VEGF) inhibitors offered a chance to add a targeted therapy to a chemotherapy doublet to see if response rates could be improved upon. Serum VEGF levels are higher in MPM than in many other solid tumors, and given the efficacy of adding bevacizumab to chemotherapy in non-small cell lung cancer it was hoped that a similar advantage would be seen in mesothelioma [42, 43]. Kindler et al. reported the results of a randomized phase II study of cisplatin and gemcitabine with bevacizumab vs. placebo in patients with advanced MPM [44]. Patients received six cycles of therapy and then continued on bevacizumab or placebo until progression. The PR rates were similar in both arms (24.5 % vs. 21.8 %). The estimated median OS was 15.6 months (95 % CI, 10.6–18.7 months) for the study arm and 14.7 months (95 % CI, 10.3–20.0 months) for the placebo. The OS curves were not significantly different. Not surprisingly, bevacizumab toxicities such as epistaxis, proteinuria, and hypertension were noticed more in the treatment arm.

Bevacizumab has also been paired with the oral small molecular inhibitor of thymidine kinase, erlotinib. Jackman et al. reported on a trial utilizing second-line therapy with erlotinib at a dose of 150 mg a day coupled with bevacizumab at 15 mg/kg every 3 weeks [45]. The results were disappointing; despite good tolerance of the therapy, there were no radiological responses, half the patients had stable disease for 6 weeks, and the median time to progression was 2.2 months.

With the emergence of pemetrexed and cisplatin as the frontline therapeutic treatment for advanced MPM, other studies have tried to assess strategies for salvage chemotherapy. Toyokawa recently published a second-line study in patients previously treated with pemetrexed and cisplatin [46]. Seventeen patients received vinorelbine and gemcitabine. The PR rate was 18%, but 82% had disease control while on therapy and median survival was 11.2 months. Toxicity was manageable. Clearly, patients continuing to exhibit a good PS after frontline therapy can benefit from second-line cytotoxics.

Other groups have looked at trying other targeted therapies. Nowak et al. gave patients progressing after frontline pemetrexed and cisplatin, a multitargeted thymidine kinase inhibitor, sunitinib [47]. Fifty-one patients were evaluated; 12% had a radiological response, 65% had stable disease, and 22% progressed. Fatigue was the primary toxicity reported and 40% of patients required a dose reduction. Correlative biomarkers were examined, including serum mesothelin and serum VEGF levels. The authors concluded that sunitinib has some activity in previously treated patients and that a further search for other dosing schedules and biomarkers should be pursued.

Unfortunately, other negative trials have continued to accrue for the second-line therapy attempting to utilize emerging targeted small molecules. Histone deacetylase inhibitors (HDAC) have been studied for their effects on reversing methylations that silence gene transcription and which in preclinical models suggested activity against mesothelioma [48]. The largest second-line phase III trial ever completed in mesothelioma-randomized patients progressing after pemetrexed and cisplatin or carboplatin to either placebo or vorinostat, a histone deacetylase inhibitor [49]. The trial was negative, with no difference in OS and no improvements in patient-reported symptoms. Ramalingam et al. published a study with a novel HDAC inhibitor, belinostat, treating 13 patients with progressive MPM following a prior regimen of chemotherapy [50]. Only two patients had disease stabilization, and the median progression-free survival was only a month. The authors concluded that belinostat was inactive as monotherapy.

Multimodality Therapy

The poor results of surgery or radiation alone and the emergence of a number of active chemotherapy doublets led investigators to combine modalities in an attempt to improve local control and cure rates. At first, radiation therapy was added postoperatively after radical surgery to see whether local recurrence rates could be lowered. Rusch et al. presented data on surgical resection followed by high-dose adjuvant radiation therapy to 54 Gy [51]. Seventy percent of the patients underwent extrapleural pneumonectomy; 5 patients had decortication and 21 patients were explored. Overall, the radiation was well tolerated with the primary toxicity being fatigue and esophagitis. The median survival was 33.8 months for stage I and II tumors but only 10 months for stage III and IV tumors. For patients undergoing EPP, local recurrence was rare but there was a high rate of distant recurrence especially in patients with stage III disease.

The Brigham and Women's Hospital in Boston has had a strategy of utilizing trimodality therapy since 1980. In their series, patients underwent EPP followed by IV chemotherapy and radiation therapy [52]. They proved that in selected patients radical surgery was possible with a low mortality rate and that delivering postoperative chemotherapy and radiation was feasible. In general, the chemotherapeutic regimens used were platinum based, although coupled with agents that would not be now considered standard of care, such as adriamycin and paclitaxel.

A number of more recent trials have looked at incorporating gemcitabine or pemetrexed-based chemotherapy backbones with trimodality therapy. Weder et al. reported on a neoadjuvant approach with cisplatin and gemcitabine after finding it too difficult to reliably deliver systemic chemotherapy following EPP [53]. Nineteen patients felt to be surgically resectable with a PS of 2 or above received cisplatin 80 mg/m^2 on day 1 and gemcitabine at 1000 mg/m^2 weekly for 3 weeks every 4 weeks for a total of three cycles and then underwent EPP. The response rate to the chemotherapy was 33%, and 16 of the 19 went onto EPP. There was no postoperative mortality. Sixteen patients received postoperative radiation therapy. The median survival was 23 months; 2 patients remain alive and free of disease at 38 and 41 months after surgery.

Krug et al. reported on a multicenter trial of trimodality therapy incorporating pemetrexed into the neoadjuvant chemotherapy prior to EPP [54]. The eligibility requirements called for a PS of 1 or greater. Seventy-seven percent of patients received cisplatin 80 mg/m^2 and pemetrexed 500 mg/m^2/day of a 3-week cycle for four cycles. All patients received vitamin supplementation. The radiographic response rate was 32.5%, and 54 of the original 77 went on to EPP. There were three complete responses. Forty of the 44 patients went onto complete the 54 Gy of postoperative radiation therapy. The median OS of the entire group was 16.8 months; those patients who were able to successfully complete all modalities of treatment had a median survival of 29.1 months and a 2-year survival rate of 61.2%.

The role of radical surgery in the management of resectable patients remains controversial. Treasure et al. reported on their outcomes randomizing patients following cisplatin-based chemotherapy to either EPP or no EPP [55]. It took 3 years to enroll the target number of patients, not 1 year that had been the goal. The 12-month survival was 52.2% in those allocated EPP and 73.1% in those allocated to no EPP. The study has obviously continued to fuel the debate on whether such a difficult, radical surgery should be pursued in appropriate patients and if so, how to better predict those patients with MPM most likely to benefit from trimodality therapy. Clearly, many patients suffering with the disease do not tend to be younger and they also tend to have more rather than fewer comorbidities. A second mesothelioma and radical surgery (MARS) trial is underway that is comparing radical pleurectomy and decortication followed by cisplatin and pemetrexed vs. no surgery to better answer these questions.

Peritoneal mesothelioma remains quite rare—only 10% of the mesothelioma cases in the USA—and there is no consensus standard of care. Patients not surprisingly tend to present when symptomatic and burdened with gastrointestinal symptoms brought on by the development of ascites and omental caking. A number of approaches have been attempted— from palliative chemotherapy to more aggressive surgical resection—with hyperthermic intraperitoneal chemotherapy (HIPEC) administration. Yan and colleagues presented their data on 405 patients treated with aggressive cytoreductive surgery (CRS) with HIPEC [56]. The therapy was morbid; the average hospital stay was 22 days. However, the overall median survival was 53 months (1–235 months), and 3- and 5-year survival rates were 60 and 47%, respectively. It is still not a consensus opinion that this approach should always be utilized; critics have pointed out that the relative contribution of HIPEC to CRS cannot be answered without a randomized trial against CRS alone, and the cost and morbidity are significant [57].

Conclusion

Improving results for patients with advanced mesothelioma has been a frustrating and sobering effort. While pemetrexed-based regimens have clearly demonstrated significant clinical activity, trimodality approaches in patients with good PS and utilizing aggressive surgery still seem to have hit a ceiling in regard to OS. Still, patients with few comorbidities, a good PS, and epithelial subtypes should be treated in centers with experience with a multidisciplinary approach. Unlike the results found with lung adenocarcinoma that have driver mutations (such as epidermal growth factor receptor; EGFR-activating mutations, or anaplastic lymphoma kinase (ALK) translocations), mesothelioma seems thus far to be recalcitrant to the development of targeted therapies. It is hoped that further advances in genomics, epigenetics, and immunotherapy will eventually lead to improved therapeutics that will benefit patients suffering with the disease.

References

1. Weill H, Hughes JM, Churg AM. Changing trends in US mesothelioma incidence. Occup Environ Med. 2004;61:438–41.
2. Peto J, Decarli A, La Vecchia C, Levi F, Negri E. The European mesothelioma epidemic. Br J Cancer. 1999;79(3–4):666–72.
3. Robinson BM. Malignant pleural mesothelioma: an epidemiological perspective. Ann Cardiothorac Surg. 2012;1(4):491–6.
4. Herndon JE, Green MR, Chahinian AP, Corson JM, Suzuki Y, Vogelzang NJ. Factors predictive of survival among 337 patients with mesothelioma treated between 1984 and 1994 by the Cancer and Leukemia Group B. Chest. 1998;113(3):723–31.

5. Erasmus JJ, Truong MT, Smythe WR, Munden RF, Marom EM, Rice DC, Vaporciyan AA, Walsh GL, Sabloff BS, Broemeling LD, Stevens CW, Pisters KM, Podoloff DA, Macapinlac HA. Integrated computed tomography-positron emission tomography in patients with potentially resectable malignant pleural mesothelioma: staging implications. J Thorac Cardiovasc Surg. 2005;129(6):1364–70.
6. Nakano T, Fujii J, Tamura S, Hada T, Higashino K. Thrombocytosis in patients with malignant pleural mesothelioma. Cancer. 1986;58(8):1699–701.
7. Pass HI, Levin SM, Harbut MR, Melamed J, Chiriboga L, Donington J, Huflejt M, Carbone M, Chia D, Goodglick L, Goodman GE, Thornquist MD, Liu G, de Perrot M, Tsao MS, Goparaju C. Fibulin-3 as a blood and effusion biomarker for pleural mesothelioma. N Engl J Med. 2012;367:1417–27.
8. Pilling J, Dartnell JA, Lang-Lazdunski L. Integrated positron emission tomography-computed tomography does not accurately stage intrathoracic disease of patients undergoing trimodality therapy for malignant pleural mesothelioma. Thorac Cardiovasc Surg. 2010;58(4):215–9. doi: 10.1055/s-0029-1241029.
9. Rusch V, Baldini EH, Bueno R, et al. The role of surgical cytoreduction in the treatment of malignant pleural mesothelioma: meeting summary of the International Mesothelioma Interest Group Congress, September 11–14, 2012, Boston, Mass. J Thorac Cardiovasc Surg. 2013;145:909–10.
10. Flores RM, Pass HI, Seshan VE, et al. Extrapleural pneumonectomy versus pleurectomy/decortication in the surgical management of malignant pleural mesothelioma: results in 663 patients. J Thorac Cardiovasc Surg. 2008;135:620–6, e1–3.
11. Sugarbaker DJ, Wolf AS, Chirieac LR, et al. Clinical and pathological features of three-year survivors of malignant pleural mesothelioma following extrapleural pneumonectomy. Eur J Cardiothorac Surg. 2011;40:298–303.
12. Sugarbaker DJ, Wolf AS. Surgery for malignant pleural mesothelioma. Expert Rev Respir Med. 2010;4:363–72.
13. Wolf AS, Richards WG, Tilleman TR, et al. Characteristics of malignant pleural mesothelioma in women. Ann Thorac Surg. 2010;90:949–56; discussion 56.
14. Rusch VW, Giroux D. Do we need a revised staging system for malignant pleural mesothelioma? Analysis of the IASLC database. Ann Cardiothorac Surg. 2012;1:438–48.
15. Wolf AS, Daniel J, Sugarbaker DJ. Surgical techniques for multimodality treatment of malignant pleural mesothelioma: extrapleural pneumonectomy and pleurectomy/decortication. Semin Thorac Cardiovasc Surg. 2009;21:132–48.
16. Sugarbaker DJ, Gill RR, Yeap BY, et al. Hyperthermic intraoperative pleural cisplatin chemotherapy extends interval to recurrence and survival among low-risk patients with malignant pleural mesothelioma undergoing surgical macroscopic complete resection. J Thorac Cardiovasc Surg. 2013;145:955–63.
17. Tilleman TR, Richards WG, Zellos L, et al. Extrapleural pneumonectomy followed by intracavitary intraoperative hyperthermic cisplatin with pharmacologic cytoprotection for treatment of malignant pleural mesothelioma: a phase II prospective study. J Thorac Cardiovasc Surg. 2009;138:405–11.
18. de Graaf-Strukowska L, van der Zee J, van Putten W, et al. Factors influencing the outcome of radiotherapy in malignant mesothelioma of the pleura–a single institution experience with 189 patients. Int J Radiat Oncol Biol Phys. 1999;43:511–6.
19. Kutcher GJ, Kestler C, Greenblat D, et al. Technique for external beam treatment for mesothelioma. Int J Radiat Oncol Biol Phys. 1987; 13:1747–52.
20. Gupta V, Mychalczak B, Krug L, et al. Hemithoracic radiation therapy after pleurectomy/decortication for malignant pleural mesothelioma. Int J Radiat Oncol Biol Phys. 2005;63:1045–52.
21. Yajnik S, Rosenzweig KE, Mychalczak B, et al. Hemithoracic radiation after extrapleural pneumonectomy for malignant pleural mesothelioma. Int J Radiat Oncol Biol Phys. 2003;56:1319–26.

22. Flores RM, Krug LM, Rosenzweig KE, et al. Induction chemotherapy, extrapleural pneumonectomy, and post-operative high-dose radiotherapy for locally advanced malignant pleural mesothelioma: a phase II trial. J Thorac Oncol. 2006;1:289–95.
23. Rice DC, Stevens CW, Correa AM, et al. Outcomes after extrapleural pneumonectomy and intensity-modulated radiation therapy for malignant pleural mesothelioma. Ann Thorac Surg. 2007;84:1685–93.
24. Buduhan G, Menon S, Aye R, et al. Trimodality therapy for malignant pleural mesothelioma. Ann Thorac Surg. 2009;88:870–6.
25. Allen AM, Czerminska M, Janne PA, et al. Fatal pneumonitis associated with intensity modulated radiation therapy for mesothelioma. Int J Radiat Oncol Biol Phys. 2006;65(3):640–5.
26. Rice DC, Smythe WR, Liao Z, et al. Dose-dependent pulmonary toxicity after postoperative intensity-modulated radiotherapy for malignant pleural mesothelioma. Int J Radiat Oncol Biol Phys. 2007;69:350–7.
27. Chi A, Liao Z, Nguyen NP, Howe C, Gomez D, Jang SY, Komaki R. Intensity-modulated radiotherapy after extrapleural pneumonectomy in the combined-modality treatment of malignant pleural mesothelioma. J Thorac Oncol. 2011;6(6):1132–41.
28. Bölükbas S, Eberlein M, Schirren J. Prospective study on functional results after lung-sparing radical pleurectomy in the management of malignant pleural mesothelioma. J Thorac Oncol. 2012;7(5):900–5.
29. Minatel E, et al. Radical pleurectomy/decortication followed by high dose of radiation therapy for malignant pleural mesothelioma. Final results with long-term follow-up. Lung Cancer 2013. http://dx.doi.org/10.1016/j.lungcan.2013.10.013.
30. Gomez DR, Hong DS, Allen PK, et al. Patterns of failure, toxicity, and survival after extrapleural pneumonectomy and hemithoracic intensity-modulated radiation therapy for malignant pleural mesothelioma. J Thorac Oncol. 2013;8(2):238–45.
31. Rosenzweig K. Current readings: improvements in intensity modulated radiation therapy for malignant pleural mesothelioma. Semin Thoracic Surg. http://dx.doi.org/10.1053/j.semtcvs.2013.10.004.
32. de Graaf-Strukowska L, van der Zee J, van Putten W et al. Factors influencing the outcome of radiotherapy in malignant mesothelioma of the pleura–a single-institution experience with 189 patients. Int J Radiat Oncol Biol Phys. 1999;43:511–6.
33. Ong ST, Vogelzang NJ. Chemotherapy in malignant pleural mesothelioma. A review. J Clin Oncol. 1996;14(3):1007–17.
34. Byrne MJ, Davidson JA, Musk AW, Dewar J, van Hazel G, Buck M, de Klerk NH, Robins BWS. Cisplatin and gemcitabine treatment for malignant mesothelioma: a phase II study. J Clin Oncol. 1999;17(1):25–30.
35. Nowak AK, Byrne MJ, Williamson R, Ryan G, Segal A, Fielding D, Mitchell P, Musk AW, Robinson BW. A multicentre phase II study of cisplatin and gemcitabine for malignant mesothelioma. Br J Cancer. 2002;87(5):491–6.
36. Chattopadhyay S, Moran RG, Goldman ID. Pemetrexed: biochemical and cellular pharmacology, mechanisms, and clinical applications. Mol Cancer Ther. 2007;6(2):404–17.
37. Thödtman R, Depenbrock H, Dumez H, Blatter J, Johnson RD, van Oosterom A, Hanauske A-R. Clinical and pharmacokinetic phase I study of multitargeted antifolate (LY231514) in combination with cisplatin. J Clin Oncol. 1999;17(10):3009–16.
38. Vogelzang NJ, Rusthoven JJ, Symanowski J, Denham C, Kaukel E, Ruffie P, Gatzemeier U, Boyer M, Emri S, Manegold C, Niyikiza C, Paoletti P. Phase III study of pemetrexed in combination with cisplatin versus cisplatin alone in patients with malignant pleural mesothelioma. J Clin Oncol 2003;21(14):2636–26.
39. van Meerbeeck JP, Gaafar R, Manegold C, Van Klaveren RJ, Van Marck EA, Vincent M, Legrand C, Bottomley A, Debruyne C, Giaccone G. Randomized phase III study of cisplatin with or without raltitrexed in patients with malignant pleural mesothelioma: an intergroup study of the European Organisation for Research and Treatment of Cancer Lung Cancer Group and the National Cancer Institute of Canada. J Clin Oncol. 2005;23(28):6881–9.

40. Jänne PA, Simon GR, Langer CJ, Taub RN, Dowlati A, Fidias P, Monberg M, Obasaju C, Kindler H. Phase II trial of pemetrexed and gemcitabine in chemotherapy-naïve malignant pleural mesothelioma. J Clin Oncol. 2008;26(9):1465–71.
41. Ceresoli GL, Zucali PA, Favaretto AG, Grossi F, Bidoli P, Conte GD, Ceribelli A, Bearz A, Morenghi E, Cavina R, Marangolo M, Soto Parra HJ, Santoro A. Phase II study of pemetrexed plus carboplatin in malignant pleural mesothelioma. J Clin Oncol. 2006;24(9):1443–8.
42. Yasumitsu A, Tabata C, Tabata R, Hirayama N, Murakami A, Yamada S, Terada T, Iida S, Tamura K, Fukuoka K, Kuribayashi K, Nakano T. Clinical significance of serum vascular endothelial growth factor in malignant pleural mesothelioma. J Thorac Oncol. 2010;5(4):479–83.
43. Strizzi L, Catalano A, Vianale G, Orecchia S, Casalini A, Tassi G, Puntoni R, Mutti L, Procopio A. Vascular endothelial growth factor is an autocrine growth factor in human malignant mesothelioma. J Pathol. 2001;193(4):468–75.
44. Kindler HL, Karrison TG, Gandara DR, Lu C, Krug LM, Stevenson JP, Jänne PA, Quinn DI, Koczywas MN, Brahmer JR, Albain KS, Taber DA, Armato III SG, Vogelzang NJ, Chen HX, Stadler WM, Vokes EE. Multicenter, double-blind, placebo-controlled, randomized phase II trial of gemcitabine/cisplatin plus bevacizumab or placebo in patients with malignant mesothelioma. J Clin Oncol. 2012;30(20):2509–15.
45. Jackman DM, Kindler HL, Yeap BY, Fidias P, Salgia R, Lucca J, Morse LK, Ostler PA, Johnson BE, Jänne PA. Erlotinib plus bevacizumab in previously treated patients with malignant pleural mesothelioma. Cancer. 2008;113(4):808–14.
46. Toyokawa G, Takenoyama M, Hirai F, Toyozawa R, Inamasu E, Kojo M, Morodomi Y, Shiraishi Y, Takenaka T, Yamaguchi M, Shimokawa M, Seto T, Ichinose Y. Gemcitabine and vinorelbine as second-line or beyond treatment in patients with malignant pleural mesothelioma pretreated with platinum plus pemetrexed chemotherapy. Int J Clin Oncol. 2014;19(4):601–6.
47. Nowak AK, Millward MJ, Creaney J, Francis RJ, Dick IM, Hasani A, van der Schaaf A, Segal A, Musk AW, Byrne MJ. A phase II study of intermittent sunitinib malate as second-line therapy in progressive malignant pleural mesothelioma. J Thorac Oncol. 2012;7(9):1449–56.
48. Crisanti MC, Wallace AF, Kapoor V, Vandermeers F, Dowling ML, Pereira LP, Coleman K, Campling BG, Fridlender ZG, Kao GD, Albelda SM. The HDAC inhibitor panobinostat (LBH589) inhibits mesothelioma and lung cancer cells in vitro and in vivo with particular efficacy for small cell lung cancer. Mol Cancer Ther. 2009;8(8):2221–31.
49. Krug LM, Kindler H, Calvert H, Manegold C, Tsao AS, Fennell D, Lubiniecki GM, Sun X, Smith M, Baas P. VANTAGE 014: Vorinostat (V) in patients with advanced Malignant Pleural Mesothelioma (MPM) who have failed prior pemetrexed and either cisplatin or carboplatin therapy: a phase III, randomized, double-blind, placebo-controlled trial. Eur J Cancer. 2011;47(Suppl 2):2–3.
50. Ramalingam SS, Belani CP, Ruel C, Frankel P, Gitlitz B, Koczywas M, Espinoza-Delgado I, Gandara D. Phase II study of Belinostat (PXD101), a histone deacetylase inhibitor, for second line therapy of advanced malignant pleural mesothelioma. J Thorac Oncol. 2009;4(1):97–101.
51. Rusch VW, Rosenzweig K, Venkatraman E, Leon L, Raben A, Harrison L, Bains MS, Downey RJ, Ginsberg RJ. A phase II trial of surgical resection and adjuvant high-dose hemithoracic radiation for malignant pleural mesothelioma. J Thorac Cardiovasc Surg 2001;122:788–95.
52. Sugarbaker DJ, Flores RM, Jaklitsch MT, Richards WG, Strauss GM, Corson JM, DeCamp MM Jr, Swanson SJ, Bueno R, Lukanich JM, Baldini EH, Mentzer SJ. Resection margins, extrapleural nodal status, and cell type determine postoperative long-term survival in trimodality therapy of malignant pleural mesothelioma: results in 183 patients. J Thorac Cardiovasc Surg. 1999;117(1):54–65.
53. Weder W, Kestenholz P, Taverna C, Bodis S, Lardinois D, Jerman M, Stahel RA. Neoadjuvant chemotherapy followed by extrapleural pneumonectomy in malignant pleural mesothelioma. J Clin Oncol. 2004;22(17):3451–7.

54. Krug LM, Pass HI, Rusch VW, Kindler HL, Sugarbaker DJ, Rosenzweig KE, Flores R, Friedberg JS, Pisters K, Monberg M, Obasaju CK, Vogelzang NJ. Multicenter phase II trial of neoadjuvant pemetrexed plus cisplatin followed by extrapleural pneumonectomy and radiation for malignant pleural mesothelioma. J Clin Oncol. 2009;27(18):3007–13.
55. Treasure T, Lang-Lazdunski L, Waller D, Bliss JM, Tan C, Entwisle J, Snee M, O'Brien M, Thomas G, Senan S, O'Byrne K, Kilburn LC, Spicer J, Landau D, Edwards J, Coombes G, Darlison L, Peto J, for the MARS trialists. Extra-pleural pneumonectomy versus no extra-pleural pneumonectomy for patients with malignant pleural mesothelioma: clinical outcomes of the Mesothelioma and Radical Surgery (MARS) randomised feasibility study. Lancet Oncol. 2011;12(8):763–72.
56. Yan TD, Deraco M, Baratti D, Kusamura S, Elias D, Glehen O, Gilly FN, Levine EA, Shen P, Mohamed F, Moran BJ, Morris DL, Chua TC, Piso P, Sugarbaker PH. Cytoreductive surgery and hyperthermic intraperitoneal chemotherapy for malignant peritoneal mesothelioma: multi-institutional experience. J Clin Oncol. 2009;27(36):6237–42.
57. Markman M. Continued uncertainty regarding hyperthermic intraperitoneal chemotherapy in malignant peritoneal mesothelioma. J Clin Oncol. 2010;28(24):e418.

Index

A
Abdominal distension, 37–39
Adenocarcinoma, 98, 101
   colonic, 96
   lung, 81, 95, 98, 102, 135
   primary, 82
   pulmonary, 99–101
Adequacy, 1, 94
Asbestos, 2–4, 6, 7, 9–16, 20, 59, 107, 125, 126
   fibers, 119
   milling, 17
Ascites, 36, 38, 39, 135

B
Biomarker,
   for malignant mesothelioma, 44, 45
Biopsy, 1, 2, 55, 60
   incisions, 70
BRCA1 associated protein 1 (BAP1), 115, 117
   syndrome disease, 18, 19, 24

C
Calretinin, 75, 76, 82, 93, 95–97
Chemotherapy, 15, 36, 42, 125, 129, 134
   for MPM, 131–133
   intracavitary, 6
   intraoperative, 128
   neoadjuvant, 126, 134
   palliative, 135
   perioperative, 21
Computed Tomography (CT), 51, 54, 55, 59, 60, 126
Cyclin dependent kinase inhibitor (CDK) 2AC (CDKN2A), 108, 111, 113

D
Desmoplastic, 1, 77, 94
   reaction, 82
Diagnosis, 23, 37–39, 41
   of DMM, 1, 2
   of mesothelioma, 16, 42
   primary tumor, 15
Differential diagnosis, 1, 2, 45, 89, 97
   of DMM, 80

E
Exposure, 2–4, 11, 14, 126
   abestos, 15, 16, 18, 20
   amosite, 8
   crocidolite, 8
   enviornmental, 6, 9
   erionite, 17
   thorotrast, 15, 23
Extra-pleural pneumonectomy, 134

G
Genetics, 19
Gross and histology of epithelial, 70, 72, 74

I
Imaging, 47, 55, 126
   assessment, 55
   modalities, 47
Immunohistochemistry, 18, 75, 81, 93
   role of, 94, 96

K
Keratin, 98
   immunostain, 78

L
Latency, 5, 14–16, 125

M
Magnetic Resonance Imaging (MRI), 55
Malignant mesothelioma, 3, 4, 6, 9, 14–16, 37, 39, 41, 42, 51, 53, 108
   biomakers for, 44, 45
   demographics of, 42, 43
   peritoneal, 19–21, 23, 24, 38
Medical-legal, 1, 2
Merlin, 113, 115
Mesothelioma, 8, 10
   incidence of pleural, 3, 4
   malignant peritoneal, 43
   malignant pleural, 43
   radiation-associated, 14, 15

P
P16ink4a, 108, 111
Paraneoplastic syndrome, 37, 41, 42
Pleural effusion, 33, 36, 43, 45, 50, 54, 58, 59, 86
   bilateral, 36
Pleurectomy and decortication, 126, 135
Prognosis, 14, 21, 24, 117
   dismisal, 1

R
Radiation, 6, 14, 15
   dosages, 14
   therapy, 129–131
Radiograph, 47
   chest, 50, 60, 63
Radiology, 95

S
Sarcoma and chronic pleuritis, 75
Sarcomatous, 1, 70, 75, 100
   keratin-negative, 97

T
Targeted therapies, 133, 135
Thrombomodulin (TM), 96

U
Ultrasonography, 47, 58, 63

V
VEGF, 133
   inhibitors, 132

W
WT1, 95, 97
   protein, 99

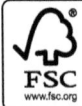

MIX
Papier aus verantwortungsvollen Quellen
Paper from responsible sources
FSC® C105338

If you have any concerns about our products,
you can contact us on
ProductSafety@springernature.com

In case Publisher is established outside the EU,
the EU authorized representative is:
**Springer Nature Customer Service Center GmbH
Europaplatz 3, 69115 Heidelberg, Germany**

Printed by Libri Plureos GmbH
in Hamburg, Germany